RENAISSANCE FOOD FROM RABELAIS TO SHAKESPEARE

Renaissance Food from Rabelais to Shakespeare
Culinary Readings and Culinary Histories

Edited by

JOAN FITZPATRICK
Loughborough University, UK

ASHGATE

Published by
Ashgate Publishing Limited
Wey Court East
Union Road
Farnham
Surrey, GU9 7PT
England

Ashgate Publishing Company
Suite 420
101 Cherry Street
Burlington
VT 05401-4405
USA

www.ashgate.com

British Library Cataloguing in Publication Data
Renaissance food from Rabelais to Shakespeare: culinary readings and culinary histories.
   1. Food habits – Europe – History – 16th century. 2. Food habits – Europe – History – 17th century. 3. Food habits in literature. 4. Diet in literature. 5. Cookery in literature. 6. Food writing – Europe – History – 16th century. 7. Food writing – Europe – History – 17th century. 8. European literature – Renaissance, 1450–1600 – History and criticism. 9. European literature – 17th century – History and criticism.
   I. Fitzpatrick, Joan.
   809.9'33564'09031-dc22

Library of Congress Cataloging-in-Publication Data
   Renaissance food from Rabelais to Shakespeare: culinary readings and culinary histories / edited by Joan Fitzpatrick.
       p. cm.
   Includes bibliographical references and index.
   ISBN 978-0-7546-6427-7 (alk. paper)
   1. European literature—Renaissance, 1450–1600—History and criticism. 2. Food in literature. 3. Food habits in literature. 4. Cookery in literature. 5. Food—Europe—History. 6. Food habits—Europe—History. 7. Cookery—Europe—History. I. Fitzpatrick, Joan.
   PN721.R447 2010
   809'.933564—dc22

2009037548

ISBN 9780754664277 (hbk)
ISBN 9781409401155 (ebk)

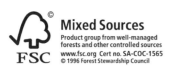

Mixed Sources
Product group from well-managed forests and other controlled sources
www.fsc.org Cert no. SA-COC-1565
© 1996 Forest Stewardship Council
FSC

Printed and bound in Great Britain by
MPG Books Group, UK

Contents

List of Contributors

Ken Albala is Professor of History at the University of the Pacific in Stockton, California. He is the author of nine books, including *Eating Right in the Renaissance* (University of California Press, 2002) and *Beans: A History* (Berg, 2007), winner of the 2008 Jane Grigson Award. He edits the Food Culture Around the World series for Greenwood Press and is co-editor of the journal *Food Culture and Society*. He has a cookbook forthcoming (*The Lost Art of Real Cooking*) and is currently working on a study of food controversies in the Reformation era.

Joan Fitzpatrick is a lecturer in English at Loughborough University, UK. Her third monograph, *Food in Shakespeare* (Ashgate, 2007) was nominated for The Renaissance Society of America Phyllis Goodhart Gordon Book Prize. She is currently writing an Athlone dictionary on Shakespeare and the language of food and preparing an edition of three early modern dietaries for the Revels Companion Library Series (Manchester University Press). She also writes the Sidney and Spenser section of *The Year's Work in English Studies* (Oxford University Press).

Chris Meads was, until recently, a senior lecturer in English at the University of Worcester, UK. Now an independent scholar, his research concentrates upon the coincidence of food, sex, and casual violence in banquet scenes from English plays staged between 1585 and 1642. He has published an anthology of sixteenth- and early seventeenth-century humorous prose, *Elizabethan Humour* (Robert Hale, 1995) and *Banquets Set Forth* (Manchester University Press, 2001) a comprehensive account of banqueting on the early modern English stage.

Diane Purkiss is Fellow and Director of Studies in English at Keble College Oxford. She has published widely on witchcraft and on Milton and the Civil War, with publications including *The Witch in History: Early Modern and Late Twentieth Century Representations* (Routledge, 1996) and *Literature, Gender and Politics during the English Civil War* (Cambridge University Press, 2005). Her most recent book is *The English Civil War: A People's History* (HarperCollins, 2006), and she is currently working on a history of ordinary people thinking about food.

Elizabeth Spiller, Professor of English at Florida State University, is the author of *Science, Reading, and Renaissance Literature* (Cambridge, 2004) and the editor of the two-volume collection, *Seventeenth-Century English Recipe Books* (Ashgate, 2008). She has published on early modern literature and culture in a number of peer-reviewed journals and is currently co-editor of the *Journal for Early Modern Cultural Studies*. Her most recent project, *Reading and the History of Race*, is a study of the impact that reading practices had on the development of early modern conceptions of racial identity.

Tracy Thong recently completed her PhD on the early modern banquet course at Loughborough University, UK. Her publications include an essay on traders and tricksters in Jonson's *Bartholomew Fair* in *Food and Morality Proceedings from the Oxford Symposium on Food and Cookery 2007*, edited by Susan Friedland (Prospect Books, 2008), and an essay on *The Taming of the Shrew* in *Desperate Housewives: Politics, Propriety and Pornography, Three Centuries of Women in England*, edited by Jennifer Jordan (Cambridge Scholars Publishing, 2009).

Timothy J. Tomasik is Assistant Professor of French at Valparaiso University, Indiana. His scholarship focuses on the intersections between early modern literary works and culinary texts (cookbooks, dietetic treatises, and natural histories). Previous publications include a translation of the second volume of Michel de Certeau's *The Practice of Everyday Life: Living and Cooking* (University of Minnesota Press, 1998) and *At the Table: Metaphorical and Material Cultures of Food in Medieval and Early Modern Europe*, which he co-edited with Juliann Vitullo (Brepols, 2007) . He is currently working on a translation of the early Renaissance French morality play *La Condamnation de Banquet*.

Wendy Wall is Professor of English Literature at Northwestern University. A specialist in Renaissance literature and culture, she is author of *The Imprint of Gender: Authorship and Publication in the English Renaissance* (Cornell University Press, 1993) and *Staging Domesticity: Household Work and English Identity in Early Modern Drama* (Cambridge University Press, 2002), which was a finalist for the James Russell Lowell prize awarded by the MLA and a 2002 Choice Outstanding Academic Title Award Winner. She is currently working on a book entitled *Strange Kitchens: Knowledge and Taste in Early English Recipe Books*.

Acknowledgments

I would like to thank the contributors for agreeing to be part of this collection and for providing it with such marvellous essays. I would also like to thank Ashgate, especially Erika Gaffney, whose enthusiasm and support as the volume was taking shape proved most encouraging, and my copy editor, Juleen Eichinger, who was attentive, efficient and patient. A debt of thanks is also due to The Shakespeare Institute Library in Stratford-upon-Avon, England, an invaluable resource for Renaissance scholars and without which many excellent studies would fail to see the light of day; the same is true for the electronic resource, Early English Books Online (EEBO) as enhanced by the Text Creation Partnership (TCP) at the University of Michigan led by Shawn Martin. The ideas that emerge in this volume have been debated and discussed at international conferences including meetings of the Shakespeare Association of America and the Renaissance Society of America and I would like to thank the organizers of these events for the opportunity to present and discuss the ideas and fellow scholars for engaging with them. I would also like to thank the British Academy for their financial support throughout the years I have been studying food and its impact upon Renaissance culture.

Introduction

Joan Fitzpatrick

The role of food and diet in early modern culture is a burgeoning area of interest, and this collection of essays brings together many of the best scholars currently working on this topic. The essays are international and interdisciplinary in their approach and incorporate the perspectives of historians, cultural commentators, and literary critics who are leading commentators in the field. Important research is here represented on a range of related topics: how traditions that developed in early modern England differed from those developed elsewhere in Europe and the impact this had upon people and their practices; how the history of food intersects with literary and dramatic art and vice-versa; the historical impetus and literary context of banqueting; the role of dietary literature (prose texts that advise on what to eat and why); and the depiction of food by writers such as Shakespeare. Also represented here is scholarly investigation of the serious practical application of early modern recipes. Here a useful comparison might be drawn to Shakespeare's Globe in London, where investigations into early modern staging practices have informed our understanding of the plays and the culture in which they were produced.

This collection is wide in scope, focusing on a range of European authors from the late medieval period to the mid-seventeenth century, but there is also a conscious attention to detail and close analysis of the texts, historical and literary, under consideration. The essays in this collection focus on the past but also gesture towards the future: then, as now, theories of food and drink and choices about eating and drinking encode economic circumstances, social aspirations, national identity, physical health, and self-worth. The collection draws upon historical data and literary analysis to illuminate the range of meanings attached to food and diet throughout the early modern period, but it speaks in a very real way to modern readers. In many significant ways, we do not resemble our early modern counterparts: we are informed, as they were not, by the Cartesian division of mind and body; and we no longer believe in the humoral model of human biology. Yet perhaps we are more like them than we usually allow: perhaps their belief in the humours has been replaced to some extent by our preoccupation with dietary disorders, food allergies, and food as a trigger for behavioural disorders. Like the early moderns, we too believe that food can be a source of disease or ill health as well as medicinal, and we believe, much as they did, that it impacts in significant ways upon our emotional well-being, which makes understanding what they thought all the more relevant.

Part 1 is entitled 'Eating in Early Modern Europe', and its focus is the cultural formations and cultural contexts for early modern attitudes to food and diet. This section considers how traditions that developed in early modern Europe, specifically France, differed from those in early modern England. Here we move from English attitudes to basic foodstuffs to the excesses of sixteenth-century France.

Diane Purkiss opens the collection with her essay, 'Crammed with distressful bread? Bakers and the Poor in Early Modern England'. As Purkiss demonstrates, most work on early modern food history focuses on the history of dietary ideas among elites. This chapter provides an alternative methodology, by examining the way food was created and experienced rather than the philosophy surrounding food. This creation and experience, Purkiss argues, underpins all of history, not just areas traditionally designated as food history. As Bertold Brecht wrote in the *Threepenny Opera*, 'Food is the first thing, morals follow on'. Through a careful analysis of the cultural significance of bread in late medieval and early modern England, the essay examines why bread never acquired the dietary centrality that it attained in absolutist France and in early modern Germany. The continuing crisis in English bread goes back much further than the invention of the Chorleywood process (using low protein wheats combined with chemical improvers and mechanical working of the dough); it can be traced to the traditional stereotype of the grasping miller, the length of fermentation required by wheat naturally soft and further softened in storage, the crushingly high cost of fuel for bread ovens, the charges levied for ovens use on manorial estates, the bread assize, and the class politics of bread. All this meant that Gervase Markham's dream – put forward in his book of household management, *The English Housewife* – of the household self-sufficient in bread was a fantasy even at the time he enunciated it. The fantasy of reviving his dream continues to this day, however. And yet the long task of bread baking was ultimately carried out not by farmwives but by professional bakers in towns, whose underpaid and overworked staff existed in conditions conducive to disease, leading eventually to labour organizations for whom the long hours required for 'good bread' were the enemy. By Shakespeare's day, bread had become the 'distressful' food of the urban and not the rural poor. Purkiss provokes a crucial question: can it be that this explains why there was no 'English revolution'?

The next essay in Part 1 is Timothy Tomasik's 'Fishes, Fowl, and *La Fleur de toute cuysine*: Gaster and Gastronomy in Rabelais's *Quart livre*,' in which the author considers the *Quart livre* [Book Four] from a series of books by Francois Rabelais telling the eponymous story of the giants Gargantua and Pantagruel and their adventures in search of 'the divine bottle'. In the *Quart livre*, Rabelais describes Gaster, the lord of the belly and governor of an island visited by Pantagruel and his fellow travellers. This episode consists of six chapters, the first two describing Gaster and his servants Engastrimythes and Gastrolatres, the next two listing the food sacrifices made to Gaster by his servants, and the last two detailing Gaster's inventiveness in satisfying his culinary needs. Critics usually focus on those moments from the text when the travellers first visit Gaster's island

and when the author explains how Gaster is responsible for inventing technology and the arts. The references to food that occur throughout the chapters featuring Gaster are usually considered satiric, an explicit criticism of gluttonous monks or Catholic ritual. But, Tomasik argues, Rabelais is actually depicting the culinary reality of mid-century renaissance France and the long list of food in the *Quart livre* actually reflects the tables of contents in contemporary cookbooks. Rabelais' work engages with Pierre Belon's *L'histoire de la nature des oyseaux* (1555) and Guillaume Rondelet's *L'histoire entière des poissons* (1558), both eclectic works that include recipes and instructions on how to present banquets as well as commentary on anatomy and animals. Crucially, far from being a denunciation of food and feasting, or an ironic critique of gluttony, Rabelais's *Quart livre* actually represents a glorious celebration of the culinary and an engagement with the numerous and eclectic writings on food and natural history that were emerging during the Renaissance in France.

Part 2 of the collection, 'Early Modern Cookbooks and Recipes', takes us into the kitchen and considers the development of the cultural artifact we now recognize as the cookbook, how early modern recipes might 'work' today, and whether cookery books specifically aimed at women might have shaped domestic creativity. We move from the history and development of the early modern recipe collections to putting these recipes into practice. The cookbook is also considered as a text that encouraged the transformative power the cook was considered to have over nature's raw materials.

This section opens with Elizabeth Spiller's essay entitled 'Recipes for Knowledge: Maker's Knowledge Traditions, Paracelsian Recipes, and the Invention of the Cookbook, 1600–60'. Here Spiller assesses the intellectual and cultural shifts that led to the related development of recognizably modern forms of both the recipe (a standardized, formulaic set of instructions for making food) and the cookbook (a collection of recipes with supporting information on the sourcing, preservation, and preparation of food) in mid-seventeenth-century England. Of specific interest are two recipe collections associated with the influential Paracelsian physician, Theodore de Mayherne. The first of these, the *Pharmacopoea Londinensis*, was initially published in 1618 under the auspices of the Royal College of Physicians and served, by royal decree, as the official text regulating the compounding of medicines that developed from the Galenic and Paracelsian traditions. The second, *Archimagirus Anglo-Gallicus* (1658), is a volume of culinary recipes that, according to the volume's title page, was 'copied from a choice Manuscript of Sir Theodore Mayerne, Knight, Physician to the late K. Charles'. The transformation of the King's physician into a culinary chef, into an 'archimagirus', offers a version in small of a larger epistemological shift that emerges out of works like the *Pharmacopoea Londinensis* and that makes possible recipe collections devoted strictly and distinctively to cooking that begin to appear in the 1650s. Spiller traces the ways in which Paracelsian iatrochemistry – a branch of both chemistry and medicine with roots in alchemy, which featured strongly in the *Pharmacopoea Londinensis* – contributed indirectly to a reclassification of the status of food by removing it from the category of physic under which it had been in traditional Galenic models of the body. The turn to Paracelsianism also brought with it an emphasis on accurate measurement brought about by the burgeoning empiricism popularized by Francis Bacon.

In Ken Albala's essay, 'Cooking as Research Methodology: Experiments in Renaissance Cuisine', the focus is on Renaissance culinary literature and the practical application of directions in cookbooks. As Albala shows, contrary to many culinary historians' assumptions, directions in the past were not imprecise or haphazard, nor always intended for well-seasoned professionals. What appears to be bizarre or incomprehensible, without exception, works when one follows instructions literally, without shortcuts and without any so-called adaptation. Renaissance cuisine thereafter becomes remarkably accessible, with its own internal logic, but no less fascinating than any other art form of the period, and equally resplendent. Moreover, to gain a full understanding of the physical experience and aesthetic reception of food in the past, one must be willing to both cook and taste recipes in exactly the same way we are willing to observe objects of art. Comprehending historic sources and, in particular, how the meaning of good taste has changed over time is impossible without the direct physical sensation of eating. Using several concrete examples of sixteenth-century dishes drawn from Italian cookbooks by authors such as Scappi and Messisbugo as well as lesser known works in France, England, and Spain, Albala describes the practice of following period recipes, using visual sources for clues, and ultimately advocates practical cookery as an important research tool. Albala also relates the difficulties of using archaic fuel sources and technologies such as turnspits and earthenware vessels, as well as procuring now obscure ingredients, all of which he argues are necessary for understanding and properly reconstructing the daily experience of our forebears.

The third and final essay from this section is by Wendy Wall, entitled 'Distillation: Transformations in and Out of the Kitchen'. Wall points out that literary scholars routinely note the ways in which Shakespeare's *Sonnets* express the durability of artistic achievement under the pressure of mortality. Sonnet 5, for instance, holds out the image of the distilled rose as a metaphor for poetic immortality and biological reproduction: 'Then, were not summer's distillation left / A liquid prisoner pent in walls of glass, / Beauty's effect with beauty were bereft'. Critics have been acutely aware of the sexualised and anxiety-ridden nature of the image of the imprisoned yet immortal flower released from temporal decay but have failed to understand that distillation was not merely a learned male practice but also a household task recommended to housewives in numerous domestic manuals of the period. Housewives of many classes were encouraged to distil as part of the conjoined work of health care, preservation, and food production. Wall examines Hugh Plat's *Delights for Ladies* (1602) as well as manuscript recipe books by women as texts that conceptualise housework as control over nature. Recipe collections and household manuals produced between 1570 and 1650 indicate that the struggle to preserve foodstuffs was not only common but also was associated with other tasks that involved the transformation of goods and flesh. Understanding the everyday practices of cookery and housewifery allows us to identify interesting crossovers between early modern literary debates about art and nature, on the one hand, and the way that people might have perceived 'lived' everyday experiences in the kitchen, on the other. With this in mind, Wall asks: Did the popular cookery books published in England between 1570 and 1650 offer women and other household workers the powerful position of using 'art' to thwart mortality and to transform, with some creativity and verve, nature's raw materials? Was there a *memento mori* of the kitchen as well as a call to overcome the march of time? Was there an aesthetics of kitchen work that we have not yet fully recognized? Addressing these questions, Wall argues that a reading of materials by Plat and others helps us to reread literary representations (such as that of Shakespeare's Sonnet 5) with a new understanding of the knowledge informing these texts.

Part 3, 'Food and Feeding in Early Modern Literature', offers analysis of the engagement with food and feeding in key literary European and English texts from the early sixteenth to the early seventeenth century. It provides critical readings of certain European and English literary texts concerned with food and feeding, including plays by Shakespeare, less well-known dramatists such as Richard Brome, and seventeenth-century dramatic prologues. All the texts considered provide an insight into early modern dietary cultures and habits, for example the banquet course. The chapters trace evidence of authors' engagement with their source material as well as the original contribution they make to literary depictions of food.

This section opens with an essay by Tracy Thong entitled 'Performances of the Banquet Course in Early Modern Drama'. This chapter explores a subject about which little has been written: the sixteenth- and seventeenth-century 'banquet course', which was the early modern forerunner of our present-day dessert. Although the practice was distinct from a sumptuous 'banquet', or feast, in that it was a course of sweetmeats, fruit, and wine, served as a separate entertainment, it could also serve as a continuation of the principal meal. The banquet course was characterized by several rituals and derived from the French medieval *voidée*, which included the ceremony of standing, or rising from tables in order for the remains of the main meal to be cleared, or 'voided'. Wine and sweetmeats were then served, as a banquet course, in a separate location before guests retired or departed. This location often boasted material accoutrements that displayed the host's wealth and usually offered a good vantage point from which the prospect of the estate could be enjoyed and admired by guests. The course would also be accompanied by entertainment such as dancing. Thong identifies depictions of the banquet course (as distinct from the principal banquet) in a selection of well-known English Renaissance plays, including Shakespeare's *The Taming of the Shrew* and *Romeo and Juliet*, Middleton and Dekker's *The Roaring Girl*, Shakespeare and Middleton's relatively neglected *Timon of Athens*, and Richard Brome's even less well-known *The Asparagus Garden*. Thong's essay also contains a detailed evaluation of how banqueting conventions were adapted to the thematic matter of the plays. Representations of typical banquet settings on stage – withdrawing chambers, elevated rooms, or rooftops and garden houses – are also considered.

The next chapter, by Joan Fitzpatrick, is entitled '"I Must Eat my Dinner": Shakespeare's Foods from Apples to Walrus'. The focus here is on Caliban's 'dinner', specifically what his dinner might consist of and what this might suggest to original audiences who went to see *The Tempest*. Early modern dietaries – prose texts recommending what one should eat and why – can tell us much about attitudes to food and diet in the period. These texts include works such as Andrew Boorde's *Compendious regiment or a dietary of health* (first published in 1547), William Bullein's *The Gouernment of Health* (first published in 1558), and Thomas Cogan's *The Haven of Health* (first published in 1584). They constitute an under-studied resource and yet are important in forming our understanding of what Elizabethans ate, how they regarded specific foods, how consumption differed according to class and nationality, and what audiences might have made of references to food in early modern drama. In the writings of Shakespeare and his contemporaries, a distinct suspicion toward fruit and vegetables is consistent with advice from early modern dietaries that these foods should be consumed with caution. At the same time, the consumption of animal flesh was broadly encouraged, although certain humoral types were advised to avoid the flesh of specific animals. We are not told what Caliban eats for his dinner, but it might well consist of the various foods that are apparently available to him on the island: fruit, vegetables, nuts, honey, flesh, fish, fowl, and eggs. What would an early modern audience have made of such foods, and what might they suggest about this curious figure? Caliban's assertion about his dinner, taken out of context, suggests a visceral creature who is only interested in satisfying his stomach, but, as critics have noted, he speaks poetically and rationally and thus presents a more complex figure than merely a compulsion to eat would suggest. This chapter considers what Shakespeare and his contemporaries, specifically the dietary authors, had to say about these foods, what the early moderns might have considered to be 'missing' from Caliban's dinner, and what they were likely to think he was better off without.

The final essay in this section, and indeed the collection, is by Chris Meads: 'Narrative and Dramatic Sauces: Reflections upon Creativity, Cookery, and Culinary Metaphor in some Early Seventeenth-Century Dramatic Prologues'. The 'cook/chef' metaphor implies a particular model of the kitchen-master's role as creator and offers us a contemporary perspective on matters of authorship, along with a possible parallel between theatrical practice and the hierarchy of the grander kitchens. One of the conceits under consideration – of giving 'the foule' to the cook to 'dresse' and expecting to 'likewise have the foule againe', surrendered but unalterably different for the addition of sauce and cooking – is not so far philosophically from the troubling figure of the wax in Descartes's *Second Meditation*. The chapter looks at the dramatists' adaptation process itself and their use of sources rendered (by the Prologue writers) analogous to the master chefs' 'use of sauces fethers'; these 'upstart' Macrobian crows all steal in order to translate, transmogrify, or 'beautify' their raw materials. A background, including a survey of the reputation and working methods of English Renaissance chefs, is also established. In addition, the associations to be drawn between stage cooks in Old Greek Comedy and some aspects of sixteenth- and early seventeenth-century poetics will also be explored, likewise the analogy made by the Prologue writers between Epicureanism and poetic taste. At their hearts, the culinary and the dramatic processes (of working raw materials to a finished and significantly altered but allied product for public consumption), have (for the Prologue writers concerned: Carew, Davenant, Jonson, Brome, Suckling) key elements of taste and consumption in common, alongside a shared relationship with the problematic matter of illusion. In both fields of creative endeavour, materials are transformed from original matter to a form of facsimile, and the preparation of food in particular has to do with the very roots of civilized behaviour (as with Levi-Strauss', *The Raw and the Cooked*), where oppositions form the basic structure for all ideas and concepts in a culture.

PART 1
Eating in Early Modern Europe

Chapter 1
Crammed with Distressful Bread?
Bakers and the Poor in
Early Modern England

Diane Purkiss

As part of his rumination on the difference between monarchs and other men, Shakespeare puts something about bread into the mouth of Henry V:

> Not all these, laid in bed majestical,
> Can sleep so soundly as the wretched slave,
> Who, with a body filled, and vacant mind,
> Gets him to rest, crammed with distressful bread;
> Never sees horrid night, the child of hell;
> But like a lackey, from the rise to set
> Sweats in the eye of Phoebus, and all night
> Sleeps in Elysium. (Shakespeare 1997, 4. 1. 259–66)

Why is the bread here so distressful, and why does Shakespeare nonetheless say its peasant eater 'sleeps in Elysium'? Most critics have read the lines in relation to Genesis 3:19. But the Shakespeare passage is toying with the Genesis reference. Bread, positioned at the end of Shakespeare's line, and sweat, placed at the beginning of the next line but one, might appear to be yoked by an assonance as well as by the biblical quotation commonly adduced to gloss the reference. Shakespeare could have emphasised the sweat by placing it first, since this is how Genesis usually runs; in the Geneva Bible, recently said by David Kastan (2009) to be Shakespeare's source-text in matters biblical, the verse is: 'In the sweat of thy face shalt thou eat bread, till thou return to the earth, for out of it wast thou taken, because thou art dust, and to dust shalt thou return' (Anon 1560). Coverdale is similar: 'In the sweate of thy face shalt thou eate thy bred, tyll thou be turned agayne vnto earth, whence thou art take: for earth thou art, and vnto earth shalt thou be turned agayne' (Anon 1535). The Bishop's Bible also is very similar: 'In the sweatte of thy face shalt thou eate thy breade, tyll thou be turned agayne into the ground, for out of it wast thou taken' (Anon 1578), and the Vulgate is identical to the Geneva version. Here too the sweat comes before the bread, causally. All the above yoke sweat and bread together in that order, and then make a segue to death and to going back to earth. This is not Shakespeare's strategy; instead, he wants to uncouple the usual biblical causal chain and create another one, while also detaching the sweat from a universal curse, death. The sweat and the bread it earns are well separated by a strong evocation of duration and duress, perhaps too well for the Genesis reference to be adequate as a gloss on the lines. The causal relation between the bread and the sweat is also inverted. Gill's Geneva commentary focuses on the universality of the curse:

> it may have regard to all manufactories by which men get their bread, and not without sweat; and even such exercises as depend upon the brain, are not excused from such an expense: so that every man, let him be in what station of life he will, is not exempt, more or less, from this sentence, and so continues till he dies, as is next expressed ... (Gill 1763, 26; Genesis 3:19)

But this is precisely the opposite of what Henry is saying. For Henry, sweat is a differend that defines the peasant by class. Why? This is the puzzle this essay sets out to resolve.

Bread is not a dangerously indigestible food; medievals and early moderns recommended it with every meal to help rather than to hinder digestion, though some did express doubt about rye bread, as Joan Fitzpatrick has shown (Fitzpatrick 2007, 53). This may have been no more than a Londoner's distaste for products seen as foreign or wrong, however, which is also Ann Fanshawe's reaction to rye loaves in the West Country during the Civil War (Albala 2002, 59, 67, 193; and see Bullein 1595, LR5, and Cogan 1636, D3R). Is the distress of which the bread is full the result of being eaten by a peasant? Does it label the bread as peasant food? This is certainly how Shakespeare uses bread to define the mechanicals in *Midsummer Night's Dream*: 'A crew of patches, rude mechanicals,/ That work for bread upon Athenian stalls' (3.2. 9–10). They are not given bread; they have to work for it. They are close to masterlessness. Bread is also the food of the desperate: 'those palates who, not yet two summers younger,/ Must have inventions to delight the taste,/ Would now be glad of bread, and beg for it' (*Pericles* 1.4.) The elder Hamlet is also overstuffed with it, murdered 'grossly, full of bread' (3. 3. 80), a line which has puzzled critics but which makes sense if bread becomes an index of a horrible class lapse, as if the elder Hamlet is now trapped forever in the very sleepy and entirely unmonarchic peasant mode which Henry V envies.

When analyzing this jagged pattern of images, critics have tended to focus on the religious significance of bread, but in this essay I hope to remind them that bread is not just a religious symbol; it is also a material object which can be smelt and tasted (Harrison 1953; Rabin 2004). It is inscribed on the body not only as scripture but also as food. If each act of eating is social, it follows that everything which can be eaten can also become a way of experiencing identity and enmeshment. Only by understanding what Marxists were once comfortable calling the material means of production can we hope to understand that registration of social identity in full. In a preliminary fashion, then, I want to offer an extended gloss on Shakespeare's line by exploring the making and naming of bread in early modern England, ultimately venturing that the distress comes not from the sweat of its eater's brow but from the sweat baked into it, which becomes a metonymic trope for all the effort that goes into bread. This essay is a work-in-progress, in part because what I have discovered is that food history connects to everything, every historical process and event. My goal is not just to explicate Shakespeare but to point to a forgotten foodway, a lost culture of masculine bread that Shakespeare's allusion partially lays bare.

The first thing to say is that most material histories of bread are handicapped by the fact that most of their authors know very little about baking, which leads to some mistaken assumptions. What most food historians think they know about medieval bread was that there were two basic kinds: paindemayn, which is later called manchet, and cheat bread, which is brown (Sim 2005, 6, 7; Wilson 1991a, 241–2). But medieval sources, including the Bread Assize (a thirteenth-century statute that set standards of quality, measurement, and pricing for bakers and brewers) actually record many different kinds of bread (Carpenter 1861, 227ff; Thrupp 1933, 72ff; Thirsk 2007, 232–3; Burnett 1989, 9–10, 236–7; Pennell 1997, 65–8). The whole notion of just two kinds comes from Gervase Markham's 1615 work *The English Housewife* (Markham 1986, 209–11). Even if we just look at flour, its colour is inaccurate as a representation of what it is. Flour is not defined by colour – white or brown – but by what a modern baker would call the extraction rate, the amount of the exosperm removed in milling and processing (Hamelman 2004, 31–5; Calvel 1990, 13). French bakers to this day assign numbers – basic baguette flour is 55, while what they call *farine de meule* is 85 flour. This last corresponds much more closely to the clear flour of earlier periods than modern 'white' flour. The sense involved is not just the colour sense, but – much more important – touch and what modern food technicians call mouthfeel. We can find hints of the importance of texture in the earliest surviving receipts (later known as recipes). Fifteenth-century cookbooks request 'tendre bread', a designation clearly about texture, not colour (Anon 2004, 109). As well, there are, as said, many kinds of medieval bread, some of which we know little about, such as wastel bread (from the Norman French Gastel or cake), which some historians equate with pandemain, but although the OED cites many references to it, these are unspecific in the extreme. There is also cocket, said by Wilson to be a 'fine white bread' and by other historians to be coarse and brown on the basis of the 1266 statute, which in a sixteenth-century translation reads as follows:

> Bread Cocket of a farthing of the same Corne and bultell, shall weigh more than wastell by ii*s*. and Cocket bread made of Corne of lower price, shall weigh more than wastell by v*s*..Bread (of a farthing) made of the whole wheat shall weigh a cocket and an halfe, that is to say, the Cocket, that shall weigh more than a wastell by v.*s*..And bread of common Corne shall weigh two [great] cockets. (Luders 1810–28, I 199–200)

But there is nothing here to suggest darker *colour*. There might well be many reasons why wheat or flour is cheaper and heavier; damp comes to mind. Moreover, the statute explicitly *contrasts cocket* with whole wheat bread (Wilson 1991a, 241). Efforts to define have been made through colour, but actually manchets (like cottage loaves in England) seem to be defined less by their dough contents than by their shape. The first printed bread recipe is not, in fact, Markham but comes from *The Good Huswife's Haindmaide for the Kitchen*, of 1594, and it stresses size and scaling above all:

THE MAKING OF FINE MANCHET

Take half a bushell of fine flower twise boulted, and a gallon of faire luke warm water, almost a handful of white salt, and almost a pinte of yest, then temper all these together, without any more liquor, as hard as ye can handle it: then let it lie halfe an hower, then take it up, and make your Manchetts, and let them stand almost an hower in the oven. Memorandum, that of every bushell of meale may be made five and twentie caste of bread, and every loaf to way a pounde besyde the chesill. (Anon 1594, 51)

A bushel of flour weighed 56–60 pounds. Again, when thinking about making or using bread, the whiteness of the flour was not uppermost. This emphasis on size and quantity was the other way in which cooks defined bread. In receipt books, loaves were very often identified by assize criteria of size rather than by white or brown, a penny bread or penny loaf.

Some bread receipts specify a shape, such as the cottage loaflike manchet shape, and this too is implicit in the receipt above. The receipt which demands a penny loaf suggests size and shape are also important. In large towns there were variants of the Assize to cover local variations in bread, and I want to look into these, because I suspect some of these bread types are actually regional variations. But what seems clear is that the kind of apartheid between white and brown is an oversimplification of a complex picture which takes little account of change.

Another thing everyone knows was that there were two bakers' guilds in medieval London, the white bakers and the tourte bakers (Carpenter 231, 295; Wilson 1991a, 211; Drummond and Wilbraham 1957, 39–41; Hartley 1985, 505). The latter are usually equated with brown bread bakers. But in fact 'the white shall bake all manner of brede that they can make of wheat', says the 1440 ordinance. It then gives a list, which includes 'cribill brede' and 'basket bread such as sold in chepe for poor men'. Which means it is no simple matter of 'white bakers' equaling 'upper class bread' – both kinds could be baked for the poor. The tourte bakers were indeed not allowed to own a sieve, but may have been defined less by this than by the ability to bake with grains other than wheat. Rye and barley are exacting, and to this day German rye bakers are specialists and often bake nothing else. It may be that tourte bakers were catering to a different kind of market or taste – or even an ethnicity or identity. What kind of dark bread you ate depended on where you lived as well as your social status, and it was not just a matter of bolting wheat flour or not. In 1304, there were 32 tourte and 21 white bakers. In 1574, there were 36 tourte and 62 white bakers. Colin Spencer sees the rising number of white bakers to mean that the public was acquiring an uppity taste for white bread (Spencer 2002, 70). But given that tourte bakers were also expanding, the whole thing may actually point to a radical decline in home baking. As well, tourte bakers may have fallen into a minority because they made some of their income from home bakers, so their demise could equally point to a decline in these enterprising housewives. The quarrels that broke out between the white and tourte bakers under Queen Elizabeth I complicate the picture even more – tentatively, it seems that ideas about kinds of bread which defined the guilds were themselves contested, so earlier portrayals have been vastly over-simplified.

A more careful look at Gervase Markham's description of bread types, seen through the lens of this increased understanding of the complexity of bread types, reveals that even his categories cannot be divided along the axis of brown versus white. The first type is often equated with paindemain, but Markham does not say this. His specifications are much more exact. He speaks of meal 'ground upon the black stones' (Markham, 209), which makes the whitest flour. These were probably imported French millstones, which were harder than English stone and achieved a finer grind. Maslin, in contrast, has nothing to do with bran content or bolting. As Thomas Tusser explains, maslin was made from a hardy grain like rye sown in with wheat as a kind of insurance against the very frequent failures of wheat. It is also possible that rye might have acted as companion planting. Seed was actually sown in mixed field-crops. Tusser disapproves because the growth cycle of the two crops is different. He says 'some mixeth to miller the rye with the wheat, / Temmes loafe on his table to have for to eate: But sowe it not mixed, to growe so on land / Lest rie tarie wheat, till it shed as it stand'. He adds that if you do want to sow them together, 'for safetie more great then you must make sure you sow white wheat' (Tusser 1984, 34).

The other large divide in type is leaven. Bread could be raised in a number of ways. Ale barm could and still can be skimmed off the top of fermenting beer, and a decline in home brewing in the seventeenth century meant ale barm was no longer available (Markham, 204–11; Korda 2002, 33–8). Once housewives ceased to make ale, they lost a supply of yeast and thereafter had to buy it – which was possible, but also chancy. Brewer's yeast was sold at markets by alewives and was carried home in an earthenware jar covered by a cloth, but there was no way of being sure it would work well (Wilson 1991a, 231, 250, 255; Drummond and Wilbraham, 353).[1] In this context, it is interesting to note that the *Book of the Knight of la Tour Landry*, an advice manual by Geoffrey de la Tour Landry for his daughters printed by Caxton in 1483, imagines a lady coming to greet a guest 'notwithstanding she had took upon her to make leaven, and withal had her hands all pasted and floury' (Wilson 1991a, 241). This is probably a corporeal work of mercy, as leaven was used primarily for 'your hind servants' bread; a receipt says 'barley two bushels, pease two pecks, wheat or rye a peck, and a peck of malt. Sieve once. Put in the sour trough. Add boiling liquid and also create a mash with remaining flour. Leave it till next day or longer, then "bake it into great loaves with a very strong heat"' (Markham, 210). This is not far from *volkornbrot* (Hamelman, 217–8). The whole thing is leavened solely with leaven; not true leaven, either,

---

[1]   The first reliable recipe for homemade yeast was given by Eliza Acton in 1845. Prior to that the perfectly serviceable wild yeast, or sourdough, had been reliably made at home for centuries and is very simple to prepare and maintain.

as it would be made now, but something much more like what the French call old dough. In Gervase Markham's compendious exhortation to self-sufficiency, *The English Housewife*, first printed in 1615, breadmaking is located after alemaking, pointing to the connection between ale barm and bread. The trouble with using Markham as a source is the exhortatory manner to which Natasha Korda has pointed so eloquently. He seems not to be describing so much as instructing. He certainly describes manchet making in a familiar way, but the receipt is so high-context as to leave out almost everything we would like to know. Though often used as evidence of a stable golden age of housewifely baking, we cannot actually deploy him like this, and in any case his categories simplify a much more complex picture (Korda, 15–20).

Because bread was so central to the diet, it was strictly regulated through the Bread Assize, which, as noted above, was a thirteenth-century statute that set standards of quality, measurement, and pricing for bakers and brewers. At the local level, this resulted in regulatory licensing systems, with fines and punishments for lawbreakers. The assize of bread was in force until the beginning of the nineteenth century and was only then abolished in London. Faulty bread was a social and ideological as well as a pragmatic threat; bread was so laden with social and supernatural significance (for which see Aubrey 1881, 163, 179; Ross 1956) that its deformation was menacing. If the assize found a baker at fault, 'the first time let the baker be drawn [through the streets] and the loaf about his neck; the second time let him be drawn and set upon the pillory; the third time his oven was destroyed and he was never to bake again' (Anderson 1923, 112; and see Davis 2004, 465–502; Nicholas 1930–33; Cockayne 2007; Sheppard and Newton 1957.)

The possible distress of bread was also connected with wild nature. Bread required the right to forage for the faggots used to fire the bread oven. The cost was varied by region but has been estimated at £40 per year in the 1540s. A decline in household breadmaking occurred in preindustrial England when the enclosure of forests and wood commons made it impossible for poor families to collect the twigs needed to fire a bread oven. The difficulty of gathering fuel spread from area to area as laws were tightened or enforced and as enclosures spread. Without foraging rights, ordinary families could not provide themselves with food. At the same time, farmers in the south stopped feeding their workers, forcing labourers to rely on the forces of commerce for their sustenance (Burnett, 27ff; Merricks 1994, 1–9; Bushaway 1981, 37; Langdon 2005; Pugh 1946). So one thing we are seeing here is the early classification of English bread as a substance made by professional male bakers rather than housewives. This oddly male bread is distressful because it becomes the cheap and poor resource of the urban working classes, precisely those likely to hear Henry's comments from the Globe stage.

What happens next is a trackable change in bread fashions, which evolves slowly in the period immediately after *Henry V* was written – and oddly allows us to notice what had come before, specifically the arrival of fancy bread, especially 'whigs' (sweet white rolls, often made with milk), and eventually the coming of breakfast rolls to go with coffee or chocolate in the early eighteenth century. Basically, women take back breadmaking from bakers. What we see is the proliferation in receipt books of many receipts for a sort of bread not included in Markham's list. This new bread, often termed 'French' bread, is the kind used in pudding receipts, which also proliferate from the seventeenth century due to the inrush of sugar and the rise of the dessert course (Mintz 1985; Wilson 1991b). The evidence is clear, but it is also difficult to interpret. Manuscript receipt books, in particular, are a problem. There is the impossibility of definite dating when it comes to the content of receipt books; they are not usually composed in a single hand, so dates inscribed on flyleaves tell us little about the dates of individual receipts. Also the appearance of a receipt even with a date does not tell us whether it was made often or infrequently or at all. How many people now have cooked every recipe in every cookbook they own? As well, most receipts are more of an *aide-memoire* than a detailed account. And finally, they obviously describe only the cooking of a literate class and its servants. That noted, here is the receipt I mean:

To Make French Bread

No 263.

Take a quart of new milk made as warm as milk from the cow, put to it a pint of ale-yeast, and a half a spoonful of salt, stir them well together, and then mix it with three quarts of the finest flour, make it presently into rolls and put them into wooden dishes and cover them with a woollen cloth, so let them stand almost half an hour, then put them into the oven and let them bake an hour (Anon, 1675–1710, fol. 68).[2]

There is a sample of this bread in every manuscript receipt book I have examined (more than forty) from the seventeenth century to the early eighteenth, and we can also find it in the main printed cookbooks of the era. Printed cookbooks of the seventeenth century do not give 'French bread' or any kind of bread at all, though they do use bread in puddings and as a thickener.[3]

---

[2]   See also Rand [1600–99?]. The recipes are from different eras and in different hands; precise dating and identification of authorship is impossible. See also Anon [1600–99?] and Davies 1684 containing receipts in several hands. Receipt books describe only the cooking of the literate; however, those who write on bread are so imbued with William Cobbett's vision of lazy housewives that they have neglected manuscript receipt books.

[3]   There is a kinship between this bread and what Robert May calls pinemolet, pain mollet (May 1685, 239). May uses six egg whites as well as warm milk, and his receipt is in the cake section. William Rabisha (1673) and Kenelm Digby (1997) do not give bread recipes, though many of their recipes use bread or breadcrumbs. Note that one probable characteristic of this bread that made it popular was its soft crust. May advises the baker to 'chip' the crust, i.e., remove it, while *The Book of Kervynge* (1508) tells the *panter* (the one in charge of the *pain*) to 'chyppe your soveraigns brede hote' (p. 5), and eighteenth-century colonial receipt books praise a 'nice soft crust'. This is in direct opposition to French practice, which favours a good crust. See Washington 1995, 113–14.

What may be happening with the rise of 'French' breads is a change in taste. Reading the old seventeenth-century receipts as a whole, one is struck by how 'dark' people's taste was – dark, slow-cooked meats, especially old meats like mutton, game, and offal, rich spicing, heavy wine and meat-based sauces, relatively few salads or vegetables. They had a taste for sourness or bitterness, as in the nowadays-none-too-edible tansies they ate, and the frequent use of vinegar. The same people were also ingesting vast quantities of homemade physic, which exposed them to another range of very strong tastes, mainly herbal tastes. Their palates were really intense. Added to which, they were knocking back a lot of very strong ale, strong in both senses, and also wine that had been spiced and sugared. Some would disagree, stressing the role of almonds in the creation of white sweetmeats, but these too were very strongly sweetened and often strongly spiced; moreover, in an era before machine drying or mechanical mills, the almonds themselves would have had a strong taste and a more fruitlike texture akin to ripe cobnuts rather than the taste we associate with them today. (Even marzipan is now too strong a taste for many, despite its refinement.) At some point, this fashion for 'dark' tastes begins to fade. The *ne plus ultra* of dark tastes is venison, which gives prestige to the others because of its associations with landownership and also with masculinity (Brentnall 1949, 191–212; Whyman 1999, 15–23), but it gets displaced by an urban, feminised, 'civilised' taste for blandness and whiteness as the acme of *civilité* and eventually health. As pewter or china replaces the trencher, shiny tastelessness replaces soaking and tasty, and the white sugared foods become more desirable than dark, spiced, bloody foods. This is probably the largest taste change ever in world history, and it only occurs in England. In France and Italy, the taste for darkness continues, though French bread does have a rollercoaster ride of brown to white to sour after the Second World War (Kaplan 2006; Kaplan 2002; Kaplan 1996). In England, it is fuelled too by rise of the potato, and one of the things that fuelled it is that potatoes are white and, as Gallagher and Greenblatt have noted, almost Eucharistic (2000, 81–112). Also, perhaps the rise of industry made whiteness more valued – darkness was linked not with forests and their denizens but with dark mills.

It is at this point that dark bread becomes 'distressful'. However, there was another source of distress associated with it. Early modern flour was very different from today's flour (Letts 1999; Wells 1988, 12–15; Burnett 1989, 8–9; Cobbett 1838).[4] Bakers measure gluten content as a percentage of flour. Strong bread flour as sold for pizza or bagels might be 12–14 per cent. Average flour – plain flour – will be around 10 per cent. Something sold as cake or pastry flour will be around 8 per cent (Hamelman, 5–13). Average English wheat grown in average English weather during the little Ice Age, stored in a barn after threshing, milled in the soft English millstones, and then stored in bins, would produce flour with about 8 per

---

    4   Studies of later problems with the wheat supply are also instructive: see Wells, 35–52, and Burnett, 92, 94, and 236–7.

cent gluten.[5] You can make bread with this, excellent bread, but it involves a *lot* of labour. Although the first detailed description of the breadmaking process in an urban bakery is relatively late for the purposes of Shakespeare studies, it chimes absolutely with the demands of the soft flour available in that era (Edlin 1992; Acton 1857). The demands of history and of ideas-led historicism may make it difficult for us to accept a source so distant from Shakespeare, but part of material history is about understanding how things must work. It literally must have been done this way or something very like this way, with small regional and local variations. The bakers begin at 2pm, do about 45 minutes work, then start work again at 6pm. Then they do some more very heavy work at 11pm – try kneading five pounds of dough in a washbasin for a sample – and again at 3am. The dough also had a sponging period of nine hours before it was even mixed up and kneaded, then a four-hour rise, further kneading, and then proofing. They took three hours to bake in the slow, gentle, cooling oven. And finally they were ready at 7am. Just in time for breakfast.

The work was heavy and tiring. You had to be strong and dumb to be a baker, went an old saying. The pace was exhausting, frenetic, like a top chef's kitchen. It was night all day, as in a coalpit. They slept in the bakeroom, because the stop-start work meant they could never get a full night's rest. The baking cellars were dungeons, often tiny, sometimes too small for the men to stand up in.[6] In *Das Kapital* (a late source, but bakers do not evolve much till the early twentieth century) Marx wrote:

> man is commanded to eat his bread in the sweat of his brow, but Londoners do not know that he had to eat daily in his bread a certain quantity of human perspiration mixed with the discharge of abscesses, cobwebs, dead blackbeetles, and putrid German yeast, without counting alum, sand, and other ingredients. (Marx 1976–81, 198)

The suppurations Marx mentions were a common feature of bakers, who worked half-naked in a hot and humid atmosphere full of flour dust. Lung diseases were also common, and so were eye problems. The temperature of a bakehouse 'ranges from about 75 degrees to upwards of 90 degrees …'. It was probably hotter still in midsummer (Kaplan 1996, 227–34).[7]

So bread made under these conditions metonymically represented the suffering of men forced to live entirely as unthinking bodies by a round of bodily suffering

---

[5] I owe this estimate to discussions with John Lister, managing director of Shipton Mill, and Andrew Whitley, author of *Bread Matters: The State of Modern Bread and a Definitive Guide to Baking Your Own* (2006). Though unreliable on history, Whitley is an excellent guide to modern bakers' practices.

[6] Further evidence can be found in Bakers' Trades Union records and in those of the separate Jewish Bakers' Union, the latter at the Jewish Museum, Finchley.

[7] Despite important national differences, Kaplan's depiction of the French boulangerie in the same era is probably accurate for London too.

we can barely begin to imagine. Distressful indeed: sleep in Elysium is bought at the expense of some poor wight staying up half the night to fuel the fires. As well, the dark bread produced by this method became an object of exactly the kind of bodily and moral disgust we find in Shakespeare. Martha Nussbaum defines disgust as 'a shrinking from contamination that is associated with a human desire to be non-animal. That desire, of course, is irrational in the sense that we know we will never succeed in fulfilling it' (Nussbaum 2004, 13). But it came to seem as if eating the 'French bread' of the housewife or the baker's whig separated us more radically from the sweaty distress of the workers who made and ate the old dark bread. Shakespeare's vacant labourer knows no night, and his brother the baker never knows anything else, leaving humanity to reach for the comfort of whiteness to disconnect us from their sweat and bodies.

Works Cited

Acton, Eliza. 1857. *The English Bread-Book for Domestic Use*. London. Longman, Brown, Green, Longmans, and Roberts.

Albala, Ken. 2002. *Eating Right in the Renaissance.* Berkeley. University of California Press.

Anderson, R. C., ed. 1923. *The assize of bread book, 1477–1517*. Southampton. Southampton Record Society, 23. Cox and Sharland.

Anon. 1508. *The Book of Kervynge*. London. Wynkyn de Worde.

———. 1535. *Biblia the Bible, that is, the holy Scripture of the Olde and New Testament, faithfully and truly translated out of Douche and Latyn in to Englishe*. Cologne? E. Cervicornus and J. Soter?

———. 1560. *The Bible and Holy Scriptures conteyned in the Olde and Newe Testament. Translated according to the Ebrue and Greke, and conferred with the best translations in diuers languges*. Geneva. Rouland Hall

———. 1578. *The Holy Byble, conteynyng the olde Testament and the Newe*. London. Christopher Barker.

———. 1594. *The Good Huswife's Handmaide for the Kitchen*. London. Richard Jones.

———. [1600–99?]. "Collection of medical and cookery recipes." New York Public Library Whitney Cookery Collection Manuscripts Number 8. Call Number MssCol 3318.

———. 1675–1710. *Boyle Family: Collection of 712 medical receipts, with some cookery receipts, mainly written by two hands: in English*. MS Wellcome 1340. London. Wellcome Library.

———. 2004. Ed. T. Austin. *Two Fifteenth-Century Cookery-Books, Harleian MS. 279 (ab. 1430), & Harleian MS. 4016 (ab. 1450), with extracts from Ashmole MS. 1439, Laud MS. 553, & Douce MS. 55*. Oxford. Oxford University Press.

Aubrey, John. 1881. *Remaines of Gentilisme and Judaisme*. Ed. James Britten. London. W. Satchell for The Folk-Lore Society.

Brentnall, H. C. 1949. 'Venison trespasses in the reign of Henry VII'. *Wiltshire Archaeological and Natural History Magazine.* 53. 191–212.

Bullein, William. 1595. *The Government of Health.* London. Valentine Sims.

Burnett, John. 1989. *Plenty and want: a social history of food in England from 1815 to the present day*, 3rd ed. London. Routledge.

Bushaway, R. W. 1981. 'Grovely, grovely, grovely and all grovely: Custom, crime and conflict in the English woodland'. *History Today.* 31:5. 37–43.

Calvel, Raymond. 1990. *Le Gout du Pain.* Paris. Vilo. 1990.

Carpenter, John, and Richard Whitington. 1861. *Liber albus: The white book of the City of London compiled A.D. 1419.* Translated from the original Latin and Anglo-Norman, by Henry Thomas Riley. London. Richard Griffin.

Cobbett, William. 1838. *Cottage economy: containing information relative to the brewing of beer, making of bread, keeping of cows, pigs, bees, ewes, goats, poultry and rabbits, and relative to other matters deemed useful in the conducting of the affairs of a labourer's family.* 15th ed. London. A. Cobbett.

Cockayne, Emily. 2007. *Hubbub: filth, noise, & stench in England, 1600–1770.* New Haven. Yale University Press.

Cogan, Thomas. 1636. *The haven of health: chiefly made for the comfort of students, and consequently for all those that have a care of their health, amplified upon five wordes of Hippocrates.* London. Anne Griffin for Roger Ball.

Constable, Giles. 1978. 'Aelred of Rievaulx and the nun of Watton: an episode in the early history of the Gilbertine order'. *Mediaeval women: dedicated and presented to Rosalind M.T. Hill on the occasion of her seventieth birthday* (Studies in Church History, Subsidia, 1). Edited by Derek Baker. Oxford. 205–26.

Davies, Mary. 1684. 'Her book: Collection of medical and cookery recipes'. New York Public Library Whitney Cookery Collection Manuscripts Number 5. Call Number MssCol 3318.

Davis, James. 2004. 'Baking for the common good: a reassessment of the assize of bread in Medieval England'. *Economic History Review.* 57:3. 465–502.

Digby, Kenelm. 1997. *The closet of the eminently learned Sir Kenelme Digbie Kt. opened, 1669.* Ed. Jane Stevenson and Peter Davidson. Blackawton, Totnes, Devon. Prospect Books.

Drummond, J. C., and Anne Wilbraham. 1957. *The Englishman's food: a history of five centuries of English diet.* London. Cape.

Edlin, A. 1992. *A treatise on the art of breadmaking: wherein the mealing trade, assize laws, and every circumstance connected with the art is particularly examined, 1805.* Transcribed and introduced by Tom Jaine. Los Angeles. Prospect.

Fitzpatrick, Joan. 2007. *Food in Shakespeare: Early Modern Dietaries and the Plays.* Literary and Scientific Cultures of Early Modernity. Aldershot. Ashgate.

Gallagher, Catherine, and Stephen Greenblatt. 2000. *Practicing new historicism.* Chicago. University of Chicago Press.

Gill, John. 1763. *An Exposition of the Old Testament*. Vol. 1: Genesis, Exodus, Leviticus, Numbers. London. George Keith.

Hamelman, Jeffrey. 2004. *Bread: A Baker's Book of Techniques and Recipes*. London. John Wiley.

Harrison, G. B. 1953. 'Distressful Bread'. *Shakespeare Quarterly*. 4.1.105.

Hartley, Dorothy. 1985. *Food in England*. London. Futura.

Kaplan, Steven. 1996. *The Bakers of Paris and the Bread Question, 1700–1775*. Durham, N.C. Duke University Press.

———. 2002. *Le retour du bon pain: une histoire contemporaine du pain, de ses techniques et de ses hommes*. [Paris?]. Perrin.

———. 2006. *Good Bread Is Back: A Contemporary History of French Bread, the Way It Is Made, and the People Who Make It*. Durham, N.C. Duke University Press.

Kastan, David. 2009 . 'Shakespeare and religion'. Oxford Wells Shakespeare Lectures, Inaugural Lectures (no. 2). University of Oxford.

Korda, Natasha. 2002. *Shakespeare's domestic economies: gender and property in early modern England*. Philadelphia. University of Pennsylvania Press.

Langton, John. 2005. 'Forests in early-modern England and Wales: History and historiography'. *Forests and Chases of England and Wales c. 1500–c.1850: towards a survey & analysis*. Edited by John Langton (1942–) and Graham Jones (1943–). Oxford. St. John's College Research Centre. 1–9.

Letts, John B. 1999. *Smoke blackened thatch: a unique source of late medieval plant remains from southern England*. London. English Heritage.

Luders, Alexander, ed. 1810–28. *The Statutes of the Realm: Printed by Command of His Majesty King George the Third, in Pursuance of an Address of the House of Commons of Great Britain, From Original Records and Authentic Manuscripts*, 11 vols. Vol I. London. London. Record Commission.

Markham, Gervase. 1986. *The English housewife, 1615*. Edited by Michael R. Best. Kingston. McGill-Queen's University Press.

Marx, Karl. 1976–91. *Capital: a critique of political economy*. Translated by Ben Fowkes. Harmondsworth. Penguin.

May, Robert. 1685. *The accomplisht cook, or The art and mystery of cookery*. London. Prospect.

Merricks, Linda. 1994. '"Without violence and by controlling the poorer sort": the enclosure of Ashdown Forest 1640–1693'. *Sussex Archaeological Collections*. 132. 1994. 115–28.

Mintz, Sidney. 1985. *Sweetness and Power: The Place of Sugar in Modern History*. New York. Viking Penguin.

Nicholas, F. J. 1930–33. "The assize of bread in London during the 16th century". *Economic History*. 2. 324–7.

Nussbaum, Martha. 2004. *Hiding from humanity: disgust, shame, and the law*. Princeton. Princeton University Press.

Pennell, Sara. 1997. *The material culture of food in early modern England, circa 1650–1750*. Unpublished D Phil thesis. Oxford. 1997.

Pugh, C. W., ed. 1946. 'Grovely Wood'. *Wiltshire Archaeological and Natural History Magazine*. 51.185. 470.

Rabin, Jules. 2004. 'Crammed with Distressful Bread'. *Gastronomica*. 4.3.6–7.

Rabisha, William. 1673. *The vvhole body of cookery dissected, taught, and fully manifested, methodically, artificially, and according to the best tradition*. London. E. Calvert.

Rand, Abigail. [1600–99?]. 'Her book: Domestic cookery manuscript in English'. New York Public Library Whitney Cookery Collection Manuscripts Number 7. Call Number MssCol 3318.

Ross, Alan S. C. 1956. 'The Assize of Bread'. *Economic History Review*. New Series. 9.2 .332–42.

Shakespeare, William. 1997. *The Norton Shakespeare*. Edited by Stephen Greenblatt. New York. W.W. Norton.

Sheppard, Ronald, and Edward Newton. 1957. *The story of bread*. London. Routledge & Paul.

Sim, Alison. 2005. *Food and Feast in Tudor England*. Stroud. Sutton.

Spencer, Colin. 2002. *British Food: an extraordinary thousand years of history*. London. Grub Street with Fortnum & Mason.

Thirsk, Joan. 2007. *Food in Early Modern England: phases, fads, fashions 1500–1760*. London. Hambledon Continuum.

Thrupp, Sylvia L. 1933. *A Short History of the Worshipful Company of Bakers of London*. London. Galleon Press.

Tusser, Thomas. 1984. *Five hundred points of good husbandry, 1573*. Oxford. Oxford University Press.

Washington, Martha. 1995. *Martha Washington's Booke of Cookery and Booke of Sweetmeats*. Transcribed by Karen Hess. New York. Columbia University Press.

Wells, Roger. 1988. *Wretched faces: famine in wartime England, 1793–1801*. Gloucester. Alan Sutton.

Whitley, Andrew. 2006. *Bread Matters: The State of Modern Bread and a Definitive Guide to Baking Your Own*. London. Fourth Estate.

Whyman, Susan E. 1999. *Sociability and power in late-Stuart England: the cultural worlds of the Verneys, 1660–1720*. Oxford. Oxford University Press.

Wilson, C. Anne. 1991a. *Food and Drink in Britain: from the Stone Age to recent times*. London. Constable.

———, ed. 1991b. *'Banquetting stuffe': the fare and social background of the Tudor and Stuart banquet*. Edinburgh. Edinburgh University Press.

Chapter 2
Fishes, Fowl, and
La Fleur de toute cuysine:
Gaster and Gastronomy in
Rabelais's *Quart livre*

Timothy J. Tomasik

François Rabelais, celebrated French humanist, doctor, and comic chronicler of the fictional giant Pantagruel, was certainly no stranger to Renaissance food. Although food references pervade the complete works of Rabelais, the greatest culinary richness can be situated in the episodes of the *Quart livre* [Fourth Book] relating the travellers' stop at the island that is home to the lord of the belly, Gaster. Lazare Sainéan, whose lexicon of Rabelais still commands authority years after its publication in 1921, has indeed called this episode a 'monument unique de l'art culinaire' [a unique monument of culinary art] (446). Rabelais's mobilisation of food in the Gaster episode is often said to be satiric. The chapters on Gaster have thus been viewed consistently as a critique of gluttony and excess. However, the excessiveness of Rabelais's so-called satire records with glee the culinary sensibilities of mid-century France. Based on Rabelais's dialogue with contemporary culinary literature, the Gaster episode in fact belies notions of satire in the sense of a critique based on irony, derision, or wit. Rather than satirise excess, Rabelais employs the rhetorical figure of *copia* in order to engage other discourses on food in the Renaissance.[1]

The dialogue among literature, cookery, natural history, and medicine situates a veritable explosion of culinary literature in mid-sixteenth-century France. It seems no coincidence that this renewed interest in things culinary arises precisely on the cusp of the Wars of Religion. The insular topos of the *Quart livre* suggests a growing isolation of religious and political factions in France.[2] However, the seemingly insular literatures of food offer a corrective to this view by combining

---

[1] For more on Rabelais's use of *copia*, see Terence Cave (1979).

[2] In his topographical reading of the complete works of Rabelais, Frank Lestringant refers to the *Quart livre* as a 'fiction en archipel' [an archipelago fiction] (1993b). For him, the logic of the *Quart livre* is an insular one whose reality 'naît de la rencontre, plus ou moins fortuite, d'un espace géographique, fictif our réel, et d'un espace purement linguistique' ['is born of the more or less fortuitous encounter of a fictive or real geographic space and a purely linguistic space'] (2002, 247).

to form a unique *assiette*, or base, around which is circumscribed both a linguistic and national community.[3] A renewed Renaissance culinary imagination thus provides Rabelais with a space for constructing communal awareness of the convivial nature of cuisine in the face of divisive religious and social strife.

The Gaster episode is a crucial turning point in the *Quart livre*. It represents the last, official island stop on Pantagruel's toponymic grand tour in search of the Divine Bottle. The episode spans six chapters, the first two describing the island, its governor Gaster, and his servants Engastrimythes and Gastrolatres. The two middle chapters enumerate all the edible sacrifices made to Gaster by his servants. Finally, the last two chapters discuss how the physical necessity for food has led to Gaster's invention of all aspects of civilisation, from agriculture and architecture to artillery and defensive warfare. The episode as a whole, and the figure of Gaster in particular, are marked by seemingly irresolvable paradoxes. The apparent ambiguity of the episode has thus understandably given rise to a wide range of interpretations. The vast majority of them are limited to the material either in the first two chapters of the episode or the last two. The middle chapters that list all the foods and dishes sacrificed to Gaster thus remain detached in a sense, both from the episode itself and from the criticism that seeks to come to terms with it.

Among the most prominent scholars, Alfred Glauser (1966) and Floyd Gray (1974) emphasise Rabelais's negative judgement against excess. Bakhtin argues that the Gaster episode moves from a critique of gluttony to a representation of the material needs of a given society (1984, 300–301). Samuel Kinser explores the carnavalesque spirit of the work but sees in Gaster only 'stomachic necessity' and not conviviality (1990, 118). Though Michel Jeanneret recognises the convivial nature of food references in the earlier works of Rabelais, food for him in the *Quart livre* is associated with excess and violence to the point of becoming pathological (1987, 96). Edwin Duval, however, sees the excessive meals of the Gaster episode as an anti-papal and anti-Catholic critique. His study of the *Quart livre* reads the meals offered to Gaster as a satire of the rituals of the Mass (1988, 132). In contrast to such critics, François Rigolot sees a more positive use of linguistic discovery and culinary poetry in the lists of food that praise gastronomy rather than critique gluttony (1972, 155). Likewise, Alice Berry lauds Rabelais's exuberance in what she refers to as 'the longest catalogue of foods in the history of literature' (2000, 106). Bernd Renner brings the episode back to satire in its erudite menippean form rather than as a critique of gluttony. For Renner, use of the farce and banquet

---

[3]   The opening lines of the Gaster episode reiterate the resonance between geographical orientations and culinary ones. Pantagruel has come ashore at an island that is admirable 'tant à cause de l'assiette, que du gouverneur d'icelle' (671) [both because of its site and of the governor thereof (560)]. The word *assiette* clearly carries a geographical connotation, particularly in the context of the physical description of the island. However, an *assiette* is also a plate for food in modern French and in medieval and early modern French refers to one service of a meal in the sense of a 'course' (first course, second course, etc.).

traditions enables Rabelais to create 'a polysemic universe thriving on paradox and ambiguity' (2007b, 184).

Based on this brief critical survey, what are we to make of the long lists of food and their function in the Gaster episode? Does the length of the list merely illustrate our material reliance on the belly or the Gastrolatres's gluttony? Are these lists simply an upwelling of popular carnavalesque spirit? Has Rabelais painstakingly transcribed 300 culinary terms simply with a view to poking a jab at Catholic rituals? The sheer number of references at hand and the striking specificity of the culinary language employed suggest that another impetus lies behind the culinary richness of the Gaster episode: a dialogic relationship with contemporary culinary literature already in full flower when the *Quart livre* appears before the public. In order to pursue further analysis of the Gaster episode, we must first take stock of contemporary culinary discourses in France.

Contrary to what a number of culinary historians have asserted for much of the twentieth century, the French Renaissance did actually have a thriving trade in home-grown, contemporary cookbooks. The medieval classic, Taillevent's *Viandier*, was first printed in 1486, but the subsequent 24 editions that appeared up to and into the seventeenth century (Scully 1988) attest to its longevity and impact in Renaissance France (Hyman and Hyman 1992, 1996, 2001). The printed *Viandier* reveals a culinary orientation quite different from its medieval counterparts: its unique mix of new recipes in an old format reveals the complex interplay between nostalgia and innovation on the cusp of the Renaissance; its recipes are written in a much more detailed fashion than the laconic style of medieval recipes; the title pages of the various editions of the *Viandier* market the cookbook to an ever-widening audience (Tomasik 2003).

A second cookbook family circulated less widely, but in spite of its formal status as a dietetic treatise still managed to carve out a sizable share of the cookbook market. Beginning in 1505, the French translation of Platina's Latin text on dietetics and cookery, *De honesta voluptate et valetudine*, circulated in 14 editions throughout the sixteenth century. The French edition profoundly transforms Platina's Latin text, inserting additional dietetic advice and specific commentary about contemporary French eating habits. Yet in so doing, the French translator maintains the problematic relationship between medical doctrine and culinary pleasure.

Beginning in the 1530s and 1540s, a new generation of cookbooks appears in France that synthesises and surpasses the innovations of earlier sixteenth-century texts. Between 1536 and 1538, Pierre Sergent publishes a *Petit traicté auquel verrez la maniere de faire cuisine*, the first sixteenth-century French cookbook entirely divorced from medieval culinary texts. Around 1539, following the success of this book, Sergent prints a new edition, expanded by 200 recipes, the *Livre de cuisine tresutile & prouffitable*. This text is then reprinted in Lyon under the title *Le livre fort excellent de Cuysine* in 1542 and 1555. Between 1543 and 1547, Sergent issues yet a third member of the family, *La Fleur de toute cuysine*, combining recipes from his earlier editions with scores of new ones for an unprecedented grand total of 478 recipes. After Sergent's death in 1547, his son-in-law Jean Bonfons brings out yet another edition of *La Fleur de toute cuysine* under the title *Le Grand cuisinier de toute cuisine*, a title that became standard in numerous subsequent editions.[4] In total, 27 editions of the Sergent family of cookbooks, from the *Petit traicté* to the *Grand cuisinier*, appeared between 1536 and 1620 (Hyman and Hyman 1992, 66–8). The large number of editions, coupled with the remarkable recycling of recipes among them, bear witness to the literate public's appetite for cookery books at mid-century and beyond. Moreover, these texts and the culinary language contained within were already in full bloom when Rabelais's *Quart livre* appeared in 1552.

A marked interest in things culinary, particularly in culinary language and vocabulary, continues after the publication of the *Quart livre* and, in some cases, in direct response to it. Surprisingly, culinary discourses appear where one might least expect them. Indeed, in a number of sixteenth-century natural histories, it becomes difficult to distinguish between what is historical and what is culinary. The botanist and naturalist Pierre Belon in his *L'histoire de la nature des oyseaux* (1555) along with the physician Guillaume Rondelet in his *L'histoire entière des poissons* (1558) mix recipes and banquet advice with zoological and anatomical discussions of fish and fowl. Jean Bruyérin-Champier, royal physician to François I, straddles the genres of dietetic treatise and gastronomic history in his 1560 *De re cibaria*. Yet, Champier expands upon both by recording contemporary food practices rather than just reiterating the taxonomies of food inherited from Antiquity. In addition to the testimony of contemporary cookbooks, these texts bear witness to the culinary impetus behind Rabelais's marshalling of food in the Gaster episode of the *Quart livre*.

The opening lines of the chapter detailing the first meal depict a somewhat lugubrious procession of the Gastrolatres before their chosen god, Gaster. At the sound of a bell, they all line up by rank 'comme en bataille' [in battle array]. The martial reference harks back to chapter 40, in which Frère Jean leads a batallion of cooks against the Andouilles. The procession is headed by 'un gras, jeune, puissant Ventru' [a powerful fat young pot-belly] who is holding a pole displaying an effigy called 'Manduce' (676, 564).[5] Behind the Gastrolatres figure a large number of servants carrying baskets of food and chanting. The scene could certainly be viewed as a Mardi gras procession, especially given that the narrator actually compares the effigy of Manduce to those paraded in Lyons during carnival. Duval,

---

[4]   For the great majority of editions in this family of cookbooks, the dating is problematic because the title pages of the first editions do not provide clear dates. Philip and Mary Hyman, in conjunction with a number of curators from the Bibliothèque nationale de France, have tentatively offered the above dating in several of their studies of Renaissance cookbooks (1992, 60–64 and 66–8; 1996, 645–8; 2001, 57–9).

[5]   All citations of Rabelais will come from the Pléiade edition of the *Oeuvres complètes* edited by Mireille Huchon (1994). Unless otherwise indicated, all citations in English will come from Donald Frame's translation (1991). Hereafter, page references to both works will be inserted parenthetically within the text.

we recall, reads the scene as a parody of a communion procession. However, what follows this initial staging is a long list of foods that may be considered the largest catalogue of comestibles in all of French literature. Setting aside the seductive criticism of excess and gluttony, the present analysis seeks to examine how contemporary culinary discourses can begin to help the reader elucidate the structure, richness, and diversity of Rabelais's text.[6]

At first glance, both lists – the first for meat days and the second for fast days – appear to be a hodge-podge of dishes. Closer inspection reveals the contours of a Renaissance banquet. The structure of such banquets is readily apparent in the menus that grace the cookbooks published by Pierre Sergent. Pierre Belon, however, offers an unlikely exposition of the French banquet in his history of birds. In the first book, after several introductory chapters that orient the structure of his avian analyses, Belon broaches the topic of which birds are most appropriate to eat. This discussion leads him to a more general description of banqueting. The title of the chapter reads 'Discours sur les principales friandises es banquets de diverses nations: & des viandes qui ont esté exquises es aprests, tant des anciens seigneurs, que modernes: & leur maniere de servir à table' (1997, 59) [Discourse on the main delicacies at the banquets of diverse nations: and the foods that were exquisitely prepared, as much for ancient lords as for modern ones: and their manner of table service].[7] Belon is thus interested in both the cuisine of Antiquity and that of his own era. After discussing the practices of Antiquity, he comes to modern times. For him, the French reign supreme in matters culinary: 'car ne les Espagnols, Portugalois, Anglois, Flamans, Italiens, Hongrois, Almans, & touts autres suiets à l'Eglise Romaine, n'ont telle magnificence en leurs appareils en matiere de viandes, que les François' (62) [for neither the Spanish, Portuguese, Flemish, Italians, Hungarians, Germans, nor any other subjects of the Roman Church have such magnificence in their preparation of food as the French]. A distinction is clearly made between France and the rest of the Roman Catholic world. Belon's expression of Gallic pride may be sheer boasting, but he proceeds to document his judgement:

> Et de vray les François ont je ne sçay quelle maiesté plus grande: car on leur sert mille petits desguisements de chairs, pour l'entree de table, en diverses pieces de vaisselles: qui est plus pour la ceremonie, qu'autrement: esquelles lon met le plus souvent tout ce qui est de mol, & liquide, & qui se doit servir chauld: comme sont potages, fricasees, hachis, & salades. Ce premier service est ce qu'on nomme l'entree de table. Le second service est du roty & boully, de diverses especes de chairs, tant d'oyseaux que d'autres divers animaux terrestres: sçachant (comme dit est) qu'il n'est question de poisson à jours de chair. Mais encor que ce soit à jour de poisson, il y aura tel ordre au service, comme aux iours de chair: d'autant que lon sert aussi bien pour l'entree, & pour le second

---

[6]   This methodology echoes the call of Barbara Bowen, for whom studies of Rabelais and food 'need to be based on knowledge of what the period actually ate, and in what terms it was accustomed to discuss food, cooking, eating, and diet' (1998, 158–9).

[7]   All translations of Belon's text into English are my own.

service, comme pour le dessert, qui nous est quasi commun avec les anciens.
L'issue de table ordinairement nous est de choses froides, come de fruictages,
laictages, & doulceurs. (62)

[The French truly have a certain greater majesty: for they are served a thousand
little disguised meats for the appetizer, each in a variety of dishes, which is more
for ceremony than anything else. In these dishes is most often placed everything
that is soft or liquid and should be served hot such as stews, fricassees, hashes,
and salads. This first course is named the appetizer. The second course is made
up of roasted and boiled meats, from several kinds of flesh, as many birds as
other terrestrial animals, knowing full well (as it is said) that fish is out of the
question on meat days. But even if it is a fish day, the order of service will be
the same as that for meat days so much so that the same service is made for the
appetizer, for the second course, and for desert which we more or less hold in
common with the Ancients. Dessert for us usually consists of cold things such as
fruits, dairy products, and sweets.]

According to Belon the first course or *entrée de table* can consist of a variety of
dishes, all designed to pique the appetite. The first course would then be followed
by several substantial *services* or courses with meat or fish dishes. The meal then
concludes with an *issue de table* in which several sweet dishes are served. This
structure is virtually identical to the menu structure delineated in the Sergent
family of cookbooks.

The number of dishes served can give the impression of excess.[8] However, it
is important to put the plethora of dishes into a medical and physical context. A
great variety of prepared foods are necessary to accommodate the different kinds
of humours that the attending diners might have. Moreover, each diner would be
able to choose only from those dishes in his or her general vicinity at the table.
The profusion of food in Rabelais's menus thus gives a false impression that can
too quickly lead to charges of gluttony and excess. Indeed, Mireille Huchon, in
the notes to the chapters on Gaster's banquet in the *Quart livre*, suggests that the
opulence of the banquet is no different than that of royal banquets organised by
Catherine de Medici around mid-century. It is important to point out, however,
that descriptions of these banquets are almost entirely based on numbers of foods.[9]

---

[8]   Indeed, Belon marvels at the number of dishes that are used at a French banquet:
'Mais c'est à s'emerveiller des Françoys, qui se delectent si fort en la variete des viandes
tellement qu'au repas d'un simple bourgeois lon voirra deux, ou trois, ou quatre douzaines
de vaisselles salies, qui sont assez pour empescher deux hommes un iour pour les nettoyer'
(62) [But one must marvel at the French who take such great delight in the variety of foods
such that at a meal for a common Bourgeois, two, three, or four dozen dishes will be dirtied
which are enough to make two men spend an entire day washing them].

[9]   Huchon (Rabelais 1994, 1577) cites a book on Henri II by Ivan Cloulas in which he
transcribes the *Depense du festin donné à la Royne Catherine de Medicis le 19 juin 1549 à
lévêché de Paris*. In it, each food item is specified by the number served: '30 paons, 33 faisans,
21 cygnes, 9 grues…' (Cloulas 1985, 246). It is noteworthy that in the long lists of poultry
and fish in the Gaster menus, there are absolutely no indications as to the number served. The
diversity comes from the richness of culinary vocabulary, not the quantity of dishes.

Rabelais's menus in the Gaster episode are in fact very different. While there are occasional references to numbers ('Carbonnades de six sortes' [six kinds of grilled meats], 'Fricassees, neuf especes' [nine kinds of fricassees]), Rabelais's menu tends to privilege specific cookbook vocabulary, a vocabulary absent from the account of Catherine de Medici's banquet. Though Rabelais's lists of food in the Gaster episode are long and seemingly chaotic, they do in fact fit within the banquet pattern sketched above. The litanies of foods are broken up by four exhortations to drink in each meal. These textual divisions follow the banquet patterns noted in Belon's description and contemporary cookbooks. Each menu is divided into four services. Rabelais's menu is thus a coherent, faithful representation of banqueting cuisine, as it can be gleaned from contemporary sources.[10]

While each banquet is coherent within itself, it is important to note that there are in fact two menus provided.[11] The first menu is referred to in the chapter title simply as 'quelles choses sacrifient les Gastrolatres à leur Dieu Ventripotent' (676) [what the Gastrolaters sacrifice to their ventripotent god (564)]. Though the meal itself is not specified as a meat-day meal, the contents clearly demarcate it as such. What is most striking about this meal is the plethora of references to fowl. Poultry references indeed comprise almost half of all the dishes on the meat-day meal. Most often, these references are for the birds by name only; no particular preparation is specified. In some cases, the list simply provides a delineation of species, with the main term for an adult bird followed by the diminutive for a young chick (number 45 and number 46: Perdris, Perdriaux). This section of the list begins to take on the character of a taxonomy, much like that in Pierre Belon's *Histoire de la nature des oyseaux*. Indeed, Belon travelled all around France and other parts of Europe in order to observe and classify the birds described in his history. Rabelais's list of fowl is equally varied and represents in effect an avian *tour de France*.

The fowl in the meat-day meal, however, do not represent all birds, only comestible ones. It is interesting to note that when a bird from Rabelais's list appears in Belon's history, the naturalist rarely fails to mention the gastronomic qualities of the fowl along with its anatomical characteristics, habitat, and mating season. Rabelais mentions 'cercelles' [teals] on his list of birds (number 68).

---

[10] Lazare Sainéan's *Langue de Rabelais* (1922) and his earlier *Histoire naturelle et les branches connexes dans l'oeuvre de Rabelais* (1921) are the only texts to seek both literary and culinary sources for Rabelais's rich gastronomy. However, Sainéan's study generally privileges medieval cookbooks. Following in the footsteps of Pichon and Vicaire, he in fact attributes *La Fleur* and its related texts to the Middle Ages, suggesting that they are mere reprints of the medieval *Viandier*. While his work is useful as a catalogue of culinary vocabulary in Rabelais's text, his conclusions about specific foods or dishes often require updating based on recent scholarship on culinary history.

[11] In order to facilitate discussion of Gaster's meals, I have transcribed the dishes, in the order they appear, and numbered each separate one in Appendices A and B. Numbers of dishes cited in the text will thus correspond to the numbers of dishes and the particular menu (meat day or meatless day) in these appendices.

In Belon's article on this bird, he remarks that 'Elle est en grande reputation es cuisines Françoyses, tellement qu'une Sarcelle sera bien souvent aussi chairement venduë, comme une grande Oye ou un Chapon. La raison est qu'un chacun cognoist qu'elle est bien delicate' (1997, 176) [It has a great reputation in French kitchens, such that a Teal will often be sold for as much money as a large Goose or a Capon. This is because everyone knows that it is very delicate]. The 'Gelinotes de boys' [wood hen, number 73] seem to enjoy an equal culinary status on French tables. Belon indicates that they are 'de plus friand manger' [of very delicate eating], which explains why 'les rotisseurs les retiennent pour les festins & banquets privez, & pour les nopces des grands seigneurs' (252) [roasters hold on to them for feasts and private banquets, and for the weddings of great lords]. Here, anatomical descriptions combine with gastronomic appreciation.

While Rabelais clearly offers a geographical tour of France by way of his fowl vocabulary, he also gives the reader a sense of the actuality of this vocabulary. This can be seen in particular in his reference to 'poulletz d'Inde' [turkeys, number 58]. According to Sainéan, it had been traditionally thought that turkeys did not come to the French table until the marriage feast of Charles IX in 1575. However, he indicates that this bird shows up in Rabelais's text more than two decades earlier (1921, 303). Champier, in his 1560 *De re cibaria*, confirms that turkeys had only just begun to be sold in France a scant number of years prior to the publication of his text (1998, 481). Thus, Rabelais undoubtedly delineates all the native birds that grace banquet tables in France, but he does not hesitate to incorporate 'foreign' ones when they begin to enter the culinary repertoire of the sixteenth century.

In the next chapter, Pantagruel asks what the Gastrolatres serve to Gaster 'es jours maigres entrelardez' (679) [on the interlarded fast-days (569)]. The pilot of Pantagruel's ship replies, and his discourse becomes the meatless-day menu. Thus, the Pantagruelians witness the procession of the meat-day menu, but they only hear the description of the meatless-day menu. By using the term '*interlarded* fast-days', Rabelais is perhaps trying to insinuate meat discursively into what should be a meatless menu. However, the contents of the menu are actually quite conservative and indeed respectful of the culinary conventions for fast days. As Huchon points out, the interlarded fast days are those that appear on the liturgical calendar outside the stricter period of Lent (Rabelais, 1994, 679, n.1). Thus, butter and eggs are theoretically acceptable, though meats of any kind are not. No traces of meat in fact appear in the menu. From this perspective, Gaster's meatless-day menu cannot be justifiably termed anti-liturgical.

What is most striking about the meatless-day menu is the enumeration of fish. Like that of poultry in the meat-day meal, these dishes only appear as names of fish, with no indication as to their preparation. In total, 104 species of fish, shellfish, or aquatic animals are listed in the meatless-day menu. The number of fish dishes is roughly equivalent to the 110 fish recipes in *La Fleur*. Indeed, *La Fleur* contains an unprecedented number of fish recipes in relation to earlier, medieval cookbooks. Even the printed *Viandier* only contains 44 fish recipes. For the specific names of fish that Rabelais enumerates in this chapter, Sainéan posits direct observation and research on the part of the author. He argues that 'Rabelais a directement puisé aux sources vivantes, qu'il s'est personnellement documenté chez les marins ponantais et levantins' (1921, 271) [Rabelais drew directly from living sources, that he personally made a documentation among western and eastern sailors].

The vast majority of these species of fish can be located either in the history of fishes by Rondelet or that by Belon. Rondelet publishes a Latin treatise on fish, *De Piscibus marinis libri XVIII, in quibus vivae piscium imagines expositae sunt*, between 1554 and 1555. This text then appears as the *Histoire entière des poissons*, translated by Laurent Joubert, in 1558. Like Rabelais, Rondelet prefers a personal approach to his taxonomy rather than relying on the texts of Antiquity. Earlier books, he writes, have not treated the subject in sufficient detail. He relates his own method by saying 'Je au contraire à grands frais ai cherché en nostre mer de Languedoc, en la Gaule, en Italie, & autre lieux, plusieurs poissons, mes amis m'en ont envoié aucuns. Je les ai ouvers, é decoupés J'ai diligemment contemplé toutes les parties interieures é exterieures' (1558, preface) [I, on the other hand, at great expense have sought several kinds of fish, in our sea in the Languedoc, in France, in Italy, and other places. My friends have sent me some of them. I opened them and dissected them. I diligently contemplated all of their interior and exterior parts]. Rondelet has thus travelled the world to view species of fish with his own eyes, yet as a doctor, he also explores the inner world of his collected specimens.

Rondelet's history of fish is clearly a precious record of Renaissance ichthyology, but like Belon's history of birds, it often appends gastronomic advice to discussions of anatomy. Rabelais lists 'perches' [perch, number 105] among his fish dishes. In his anatomical discussion of the same fish, Rondelet adds both a dietetic comment and a recipe for it. He writes 'Le brouet d'icelle mollist le ventre ell'est bonne couverte de farine é fricassée en la poele, ou rostie sur le gril, non pas boullie' (1558, 157) [The stew of this one softens the stomach; it is good covered with flour and fried in a pan, or roasted on the grill, not boiled]. Rondelet is actually much more verbose about the bream which Rabelais includes on his list as well (number 103, 'dorades'). For Rondelet, it is good 'bouillie en eau é vin, comme on fait en France' [boiled in water and wine as is done in France], but it is equally good in a variety of other ways. It can be grilled after placing fennel and rosemary in its belly; it can be roasted or served cold; or can even be baked in a crust. If the salted variety is made with must sauce, vinegar, and onions, 'est trouvée fort bonne en Languedoc. Le moust lui adoucit fort la saleure, le vinaigre lui donne une pointe plaisante, l'ognon lui donne bonne odeur' (111) [it is considered very good in the Languedoc. The must greatly reduces the saltiness, the vinegar gives it a pleasant note, the onion gives it a good smell]. Not only has Rondelet given us a series of potential recipes for this fish but he has also revealed some regional culinary preferences. As a doctor who studied at the University of Montpellier, he was undoubtedly familiar with taste preferences in the Languedoc.

In terms of Rabelais's veritable catalogue of fish in Gaster's meatless-day menu, we have noted that most of them appear without any indication as to their preparation. In the Sergent family of cookbooks, many fish dishes are prepared with butter. This is a striking innovation in regards to medieval practice, where fish is almost never prepared as such. While butter may not be directly associated with mentions of fish in Gaster's menu, it is still very present in the meal as a whole. It is referred to, by name, on three separate occasions throughout the list of foods. Butter is in fact the third item on the list, 'beurre frays' [fresh butter]. A particular kind of butter shows up, near the end of the meal, in the reference to 'Beurre d'Amendes' [almond butter, number 128]. This dish is immediately followed by another for 'Neige de beurre' [Butter snow, number 129]. Frame was unable to trace the name of this dish to any known source, but an analogous recipe can be found in the *Livre de cuisine*.[12] Butter never appears in the meat-day menu, and yet it appears at least three times in the meatless-day menu. By including so many references to butter in his meatless-day menu, Rabelais was simply ratifying an association between fish and butter that had already been established by contemporary cookbooks.

Beyond the catalogue of fishes and fowl, Rabelais regales the reader with a multitude of specific dishes whose names are not fantastical creations but actual dishes that can be traced to contemporary cookbooks. Some of these dishes represent 'classics' that had been in circulation since the fourteenth century. The dish for 'canard à la dodine' in the meat-day menu (number 62) appears in the manuscripts of the *Viandier*, in the printed *Viandier*, as well as in the Sergent family of cookbooks. Other dishes, however, represent particular contemporary tastes. The 'Pastez à la saulse chaulde' (number 35) is a dish that is absent from all medieval cookbooks except for the printed *Viandier*. It is also absent from the *Petit traicté* but appears in all the other members of the Sergent family of cookbooks. As such, Rabelais would have had access to the recipe title either in a printed *Viandier* in circulation or in one of the Sergent cookbooks.

In the *Livre de cuisine*, this pastry is made by layering sliced beef tongue and chopped fat. After it is half-baked in the oven, the 'saulce chaude' is added and the baking is then completed. In *La Fleur*, virtually the same recipe appears, but later in the text, a recipe for 'saulce chaude' is added.[13] *La Fleur* also adds a second recipe for this type of pastry using beef shoulder instead of tongue. It specifies that the beef should be sliced 'par belles pieces de la grandeur de vostre paulme' [in nice slices the size of your palm]. Such details about the main ingredient in a recipe are often absent from medieval texts. Their presence in the *Fleur* suggests that the

---

[12]   A recipe for 'Naige contrefaict' appears in the *Livre de cuisine*. It is a concoction of milk, egg whites, rice flower, and sugar that is whipped together 'comme beurre' [like butter]. This recipe is then followed by one simply called 'butter', which seems to be something akin to clarified butter. Rabelais has perhaps conflated the two recipes in his dish of 'Neige de beurre'.

[13]   *La Fleur* also adds a second recipe for 'pasté a la saulce chaude', which seems closer to the printed *Viandier* version. Instead of beef tongue, beef shoulder is used; in the printed *Viandier*, tenderloin is specified. Both recipes privilege clove as a spice among others, but the *Fleur* recipe includes sage at the end, an ingredient absent from the *Viandier* recipe.

Sergent family of cookbooks subscribes to the writing style of the printed *Viandier* in which specific instructions take the place of medieval laconic recipe writing style. By specifying this recipe on his menu, Rabelais has privileged contemporary cooking practices and writing styles over their medieval counterparts.

Rabelais's familiarity with contemporary culinary vocabulary is further illustrated by his choice of the dish 'Pieces de boeuf royalles' (number 78). Admittedly, the name of this dish does not appear in any medieval cookery collections, or even in the printed *Viandier*. The title as it appears in Rabelais's menu is not actually included the Sergent family of cookbooks, but the term 'royalle' does appear in a particular sauce known only to this group of cookbooks. The *Petit traicté* and the *Livre de cuisine* offer a recipe for a 'saulce realle'. Though *La Fleur* gives the same recipe for a 'saulce realle', it mentions 'saulce royalle' in one of its first menus. In the 1576 edition of the *Grand cuisinier*, the actual recipe appears under the heading 'saulce royalle'. The recipes are identical in each text, but for the purposes of illustration, it suffices to transcribe the recipe from *La Fleur*:

> Saulce realle. Prenez vin vermeil et vinaigre autant de lun comme de lautre, canelle entiere, cloux de giroffle et sucre, et boutez tout bouillir en un beau pot jusques quil soit diminue quasi de la moytie…

> [Royal sauce. Take red wine and vinegar, an equal amount of each, whole cinnamon, clove and sugar, and put it all in a nice pot to boil until it is reduced almost by half…]

Ultimately, this recipe is a relatively simple one, with a restrained number of ingredients, particularly the spices. It is noteworthy that the cinnamon is to remain whole, while in most sauce recipes, spices are supposed to be ground up with a mortar and pestle. Instead of being thickened with toasted bread, a veritable *sine qua non* of medieval sauce recipes, this sauce will be thickened by reducing it. Reducing sauces and producing essences is a common trait in seventeenth-century cuisine, so its evocation in the Sergent family of cookbooks marks a clear break with medieval sauce practices and anticipates characteristics of classical French haute cuisine. Rabelais's inclusion of a dish endowed with the same 'royal' moniker suggests his preference for contemporary culinary tastes and practices.

Rabelais displays his alliance with contemporary cuisine in his enumeration of pâtés. An impressive number of references are made to 'pâtés' in the meat-day menu, totalling 13 in all. Though the printed *Viandier* is not the first French cookbook to offer recipes for pâtés (several can be found in the medieval *Ménagier de Paris*; Brereton and Ferrier 1981, Pichon, 1846), it lists an unprecedented number of 35 different types (including fish versions). These recipes are entirely absent from the manuscript versions of the text. Nine recipes for pâtés appear in the French *Platina*. *La Fleur* reasserts their presence at mid-century by offering recipes for 22, 19 of which refer to meat pâtés. These cookbooks attest to a significant rise in the popularity and variety of pâtés in Renaissance France. Among those which figure on Rabelais's menu, at least half can be traced directly either to the printed *Viandier* or *La Fleur*. By including so many pâtés on his meat-day menu, Rabelais is clearly exemplifying the vogue for such dishes in sixteenth-century France.

Other types of 'pastries' figure in the meat-day menu, some of which are of the 'classic' varieties inherited from the Middle Ages but others that seem to figure in the culinary preoccupations of Renaissance France. Rabelais mentions 'Brides à veaux' (number 131), in the last course of the meat-day meal, a pastry that was clearly well known in the Middle Ages (Sainéan 1921, 428), but whose recipe does not appear until the sixteenth century in the *Livre de cuisine* ('Brideaulx a veaulx'). In terms of other pastries, we find 'Tourtes de seize façons' (number 133) and 'Tartres vingt sortes' (number 144). While we find a handful of recipes for tarts in medieval texts such as the *Ménagier*, the printed *Viandier* gives the most detailed recipes for such dishes. Moreover, Platina takes pains to describe the differences between 'tourtes' and 'tartres', a distinction that for him reveals a growing gastronomic gluttony with French origins. He explains that 'tourtes' were named by the Ancients because they were made with vegetables and greens that were 'twisted' and 'torn up' before being baked in a crust. Now, he says, they are referred to as 'tarts' because the vegetables have been replaced by meats. Diners' 'gueules delicieuses demandent a present et veulent avoir tartres de toutes sortes et façons doyseaulx' (1505, lxxviii) [delicious gullets presently demand and wish to have tarts made with all kinds of birds]. Moreover, this desire seems to be French in origin because Platina attributes the name *tartre* to the French. Instead of calling them *tourtes*: 'Tartres doncques ou soyent pictagorees ou francoyses doresenavant les appellerons' [We will thus call them tarts from now on, whether Pythagorean or French]. In addition to the number of tart recipes that Platina offers, a significant number of recipes for *boignetes* [fritters] appear. Indeed, all of book nine is devoted to recipes for fritters. The emphasis on this dish may be the impetus behind Rabelais's insertion of 'Beuignetz' (number 132) at the same point in the menu as the tarts and *tourtes*.

Near the end of this profusion of dishes in the meat-day meal, Rabelais also includes a number of items containing sugar. The menu offers an impressive array of 'Confictures seiches et liquides soixante et dixhuyt especes' [Dry and liquid preserves, seventy-eight species, number 146], 'Dragée, cent couleurs' [Sweetmeats, a hundred colours, number 147], and 'Mestier au sucre fin' [Wafer with fine sugar, number 149]. The latter item was a traditional accompaniment to the sugar-sweetened hippocras [mulled wine], a beverage that figures earlier in this particular course (number 141). Rabelais specifies that it be 'Hippocras rouge et vermeil'. As such, the banquet opens with a white hippocras aperitif and appropriately closes with a digestive red hippocras. Like the hippocras itself, the abundance of sugar at the end of the meal clearly has a dietetic rationale behind it. According to contemporary dietetic texts, and Platina in particular, sugar held supreme status as an aid to digestion. Sugar also reaches its apex in the recipes of the Sergent family of cookbooks. However, as the sixteenth century progresses, sugar begins to lose its highly praised status. In Champier's 1560 *De re cibaria*, the royal physician complains of the immoderate and random use of sugar in all types of dishes.[14] Sugar will continue to fall from favour in the seventeenth century, given the marked reduction in its appearance in cookbooks from the Classical Age. As such, Rabelais's meat-day menu is an accurate portrait of the status of sugar in mid-sixteenth-century France before it is swept under the rug in the seventeenth century.

Though Rabelais's meatless menu still follows the pattern of a banquet, the number of specifically named dishes is more restrained than in the meat-day menu. The menus begin with a number of salted fish that would be appropriate for stimulating both the appetite and the desire to drink.[15] A similar series of salted meats occupied the second course of the meat-day menu. Otherwise, the vast majority of dishes listed in the meatless days refer to fish by name of species alone. Some of the specific dishes in the meatless meal such as 'purées de poys' [pea soup, number 4] and 'saulgrenees de febves' [Bean and onion porridge, number 12] are clearly classic dishes that appear in virtually every French cookbook since the fourteenth century. Others such as the 'huyctres en escalle' [Oysters in the shell, number 22] do not appear until the sixteenth century. Oysters often appear in the form of stews in the Middle Ages, but not served on the half shell. The *Petit traicté* lists a dish for 'les huytres escallees' that has them shelled and sautéed in butter. In the *Livre de cuisine* and *La Fleur*, an additional recipe appears for 'huytres en escaille' and 'hustres a lescaille', respectively. Both recipes involve obtaining very fresh oysters, opening them up, dropping in a bit of butter and pepper, and then placing them on top of hot coals. The cooking kills the live oyster and produces the finished dish. Clearly, Rabelais's reference was for the latter variety, in which they are cooked and served in the shell.

Rabelais also offers the reader a variety of salads in the first course of the meal. Indeed, he mentions 'cent diversitez' [a hundred varieties], but then actually lists only seven specific ones. Salads were thought to sharpen the appetite at the beginning of a meal, but Champier cautions the reader about excess consumption. For him, they must be eaten 'non comme aliment, mais comme médicine' (1998,

---

[14]   Champier writes: 'Sur le plan strictement médical, nous déclarons qu'à notre époque, nous faisons un usage excessif du sucre sur nos tables, et que certains aliments sont excellents naturellement. Il ne faut pas écouter ceux qui prétendent qu'on doit masquer la saveur des aliments sous la douceur du sucre. Des milliers de peuples vivent confortablement sans sucre' (1998, 335) [On the strictly medical level, we declare that in our time we make excessive use of sugar on our tables and that certain foods are excellent naturally. We should not listen to those who claim that the flavor of foods must be masked by the sweetness of sugar. Thousands of people live comfortably without sugar].

[15]   Champier confirms this belief: 'Aujourd'hui aussi on croit qu'elles [salaisons] sont apéritives et donnent soif: aussi on les sert-on au début du repas. Ainsi, on voit que le sel se dissout pour donner des saveurs en tous genres au palais' (1998, 338) [At present we also believe that they [salted foods] are aperitifs and make one thirsty: thus they are served at the beginning of the meal. As such, the salt is thought to dissolve to give flavors of all kinds to the palate].

276) [not as a food, but as a medicine]. We recall that Gargantua, Pantragruel's father, ate six pilgrims who had inadvertently ended up in his salad. The giant had prepared lettuce with oil, vinegar, and salt and had eaten it 'pour soy refraischir davant souper' (104) [as a pick-me-up before dinner (88)]. The 'Memoire' from the Sergent family of cookbooks, a sort of meta-menu, lists a number of salads, among them one for a 'salade de hobelon'. Rabelais lists this particular one among the salads chosen for the meatless-day meal (number 14). Champier remarks that the Belgians use hops for making their beer, but they eat the young stems like asparagus, in a salad with oil and vinegar (1998: 302). Rabelais also mentions a salad made with a particular kind of mushroom (number 17): 'aureilles de Judas, (c'est une forme de funges issans des vieulx Suzeaulx) [Jess's ears (that's a kind of fungus that grows out of old elder trees)].[16] This particular dish stands out among the others because of the detailed provenance of the mushroom.

In the second course of the meatless-day meal, the most specific dish is for 'lamproyes a saulce d'Hippocras' (number 23). Many recipes exist using this spiced wine as a sauce (even for fruit dishes), but none exist incorporating hippocras with lamprey. This fish does form the basis of many other dishes, and it was considered popular banquet fare. The *Fleur* includes four recipes for lamprey and one for a particular sauce associated with it. Champier points out that the condiments used to prepare lamprey are often more expensive than the lamprey itself. He further adds an anecdote about how a particular dish for lamprey, capons with lamprey attached, caused stomach pains in the diners who ate them. He adds rather cynically that

> Il ne faut donc pas s'étonner que davantage de gens périssent par l'alimentation que par le glaive, car aucune loi ne punit la gourmandise, et seuls les cuisiniers peuvent tuer les gens, non seulement en toute impunité, mais en en retirant une grande gloire (618).

> [One should not be surprised that more people die from food than from the sword, for no law punishes gluttony, and only cooks can kill people, not only with complete impunity, but also in receiving great glory from doing so.]

Perhaps by offering a dish of lamprey with hippocras sauce, Rabelais was attempting to attenuate the lamprey's association with gluttony. As a recognised medical digestive drink, hippocras certainly carries a dietetic charge. Indeed, Rondelet, in his history of fishes, glosses the highly dietetic French Platina as a vital source of information on the lamprey. He writes: 'Quant est de la bonté de la Lamproie, de la sauce, é de la grande estime qu'on en fait, il en faut lire Platine' (1558: 313) [As for the goodness of the lamprey, of its sauce, and of the great esteem with which it is held, one must read what Platina has to say]. However, Rondelet also tells a somewhat fantastical story about lamprey. According to sailors, the lamprey is

---

[16]   The 'aureilles de Judas', which Frame translates as 'Jess's ears', are perhaps more commonly known as the Jew's Ear or Judas's ear mushroom (Auricularia auricula-judae).

capable of stopping ships at sea by clamping its enormous mouth onto the hull of the boat. Though this is clearly a fantastic tale, it is intriguing that after leaving Gaster's island, the boat remains stopped, ostensibly for lack of wind.

Before taking leave of Gaster's menu, it is important to note the rich vocabulary for egg dishes, a perennial proteinous favourite on non-Lenten fast-days. Rabelais mentions eight specific egg dishes (numbers 113–20) with names that one would generally not find in the *Larousse gastronomique*: 'oeufz fritz, perduz, suffocquez, estuvez, trainnez par les cendres, jectez par la cheminee, barbouillez, gouildronnez' [Eggs fried, lost, stifled, steamed, dragged through the ashes, thrown down the chimney, jumbled, calked (572); Vicaire 1890]. For the second item on the list, Frame refers to it as an 'unexplained way of cooking eggs' (902, n.5). In his study of Rabelais's languages, Rigolot makes brief reference to these egg dishes, subtly mocking Rabelais's 'façon fantaisiste de les cuisinier' (1972: 156). Though it is certainly tempting to regard these strangely monnikered dishes as fantastical, cookbook evidence suggests that Rabelais did not in fact have his tongue in cheek. The printed *Viandier* offers a genuine, though complicated, recipe for 'oeufz rostis en la broche' [eggs roasted on the spit]. *La Fleur* lists 11 egg dishes, among them three variants for 'oeufs perduz'. The French Platina offers 15 egg recipes whose names mirror Rabelais's vocabulary: among them figure such gems as 'oeufs agitez et batus' [scrambled eggs], 'oeufs boullis' [boiled eggs], 'oeufs rompus et decoupez' [broken and sliced eggs], 'oeufs cuycte en la broche' [eggs cooked on a spit], and 'oeufs cuyctes soubz les cendres' [eggs cooked under the ashes]. For the latter, a small hole is pierced in the shell, and the egg is then placed on the coals of the fire to cook. This is slightly less fantastical than Frame's translation as eggs 'thrown down the chimney'. Rabelais's last egg dish, 'oeufz gouildronnez' does not appear in any contemporary cookbooks, but Cotgrave (1611) glosses 'oeufs goderonnez whose white, and yolk are beaten together with a little verjuice'. Champier corroborates the use of verjuice in egg dishes, adding that they are also often prepared with vinegar and sorrel juice (486). Given the evidence of medieval and Renaissance cookbooks, dietetic texts, and lexicography, these various egg dishes are certainly not fantastical.

As we have seen thus far, the Gaster episode is much more than a satire of the excesses of the table. Yet, it might be considered a satire in the etymological sense of a mixed dish. Culinary discourses from numerous contemporary sources are stewed and steeped together in Rabelais's complex monument to Renaissance gastronomy. However, this unique mixture exists only on the level of discourse; it is ultimately a cuisine of words. Returning to Belon's Gallic pride in Renaissance cuisine, we can see that his interest in matters culinary is primarily a linguistic one. He writes:

> apres avoir escrit les mets des anciens, extraicts de leurs livres, mettrons encor les nostres, selon qu'on les sert communement à la maniere Françoyse, selon que l'avons extrait d'un petit livret intitulé, Le memoire pour faire un escriteau pour un banquet, nous avons pensé meriter pouvoir estre inseré en cest endroit, pour la diversité des noms Francoys qu'on y trouve. (1997: 64)

[after having written down the dishes of the ancients, excerpted from their books, let us put down our own as they are commonly served in the French manner according to what we have excerpted from a little booklet entitled 'The Memoir for writing a menu for a banquet'. We thought it deserves to be inserted at this point for the diversity of French names found in it.]

Belon reveals his lexicographical interest by referring to the 'diversity of French names' in the cited list. Though Belon's work implies reference to the authorities of Antiquity, he discovers in humanistic fashion that Antiquity cannot account for the linguistic diversity of his own native French. Following this statement, Belon cites in its entirety the little booklet called 'Le memoire pour faire un escriteau pour un banquet'. This dizzyingly long list of foods was originally published in the *Petit traicté*, the pioneering cookbook published by Sergent around 1539. His meta-menu was subsequently reprinted in all the other members of the same cookbook family, including *La Fleur de toute cuysine*. The 'Memoire' is in effect a master list of potential dishes for composing a banquet. Yet, the emphasis here is on writing the 'escriteau' [menu] for a banquet, not on actually doing the necessary cooking. The list may seem excessive, much like the Gaster episode, but the presumption is that a choice will be made from among the many possibilities. As in an actual banquet, one does not eat from every dish. A diner is limited to those dishes within reach at the table. A wide selection of dishes alone thus does not make gluttony a foregone conclusion.

Moreover, *écriteaux* figure in another source for Rabelais's *Quart livre*. Frank Lestringant has analyzed how Rabelais used a 1538 text called the *Disciple de Pantagruel* as an inspiration for the culinary inflection of the voyages in the *Quart livre* (Lestringant 2002: 232–8). The *Disciple* itself took its inspiration from Rabelais's earlier texts, though the only other traits that this work shares with Rabelais's work are the name of the character Panurge and the theme of maritime voyages. In several episodes from the *Disciple*, the travellers encounter a culinary paradise, a true land of Cockaigne. One island is a veritable paradise of pastries and pâtés that is protected from invasion by a ring of ovens whose rears face the sea and whose doors open onto the interior of the island. The ovens are constantly lit and capable of producing pastries on demand. Yet, the pastries also exist as words:

Il y a sur la guelle de chascun four ung escripteau en grosse lettre, qui faict mention de la sorte dont sont les pastez, & de quoy, affin qu'on sache mieulx choisir ceulx qu'on veult prendre pour manger avec la foyre à boyre (Demerson 1982, 70).

[There is on the gullet of each oven a plaque in large letters that indicates the type and what they are made of so that one can know how to better choose those that one wishes for eating during the drink fest.]

Food on this island is not simply presented as a cornucopia of excess and fantastical abundance. Choices are to be made. These choices are inevitably based on how one reads the name of a particular dish.

Though the 'Memoire' from the Sergent family of cookbooks certainly operates in a fashion similar to Rabelais's menu in the Gaster episode, and many dishes grace both lists, they are not identical. Belon follows his citation of the 'Memoire' by saying that he knows of another source for culinary vocabulary that is just as rich. He writes:

> Nous n'avons entreprins nommer tout ce qu'on pourroit bien nombrer en les mets des festins, toutefois que qui le voudroit lire, le trouvera au quatriesme de Pantagruel, au lieu ou il parle des gastrolates. Quant à nostre part, nous estimons que les autres nations ne sçauroyent tant nommer de mets en leur langue que les Françoys (1997: 65).

> [We have not undertaken to name everything that can possibly be reckoned in the dishes of feasts, although, whoever would wish to read it will find it in the fourth book of Pantagruel in the place where the Gastrolatres are mentioned. As for our part, we feel that other nations could not name as many dishes in their languages as the French can.]

Rabelais's *Quart livre* thus becomes a directly cited point of reference for culinary vocabulary in Belon's natural history. Rabelais's menu in the Gaster episode, already a compilation of many culinary sources, has become the source for yet another reflection on cuisines, tastes, and words. As such, the cookbook 'Memoire', Belon's natural history, and Rabelais's 'fantastic' tale merge to form a shared sense of culinary consciousness. This consciousness is a particularly French one. As Belon puts it, only the French could come up with so many names for dishes, a tendency that distinguishes them from other nations. Culinary literature thus opens a space in which to inscribe a national identity in Renaissance France.

In light of contemporary culinary discourses, a comparative analysis of the menus at the heart of the Gaster episode reveals Rabelais's profound engagement with contemporary culinary languages and tastes. The richness and specificity of these chapters resonate powerfully with an ever-widening circulation of a new generation of French culinary literature. In its codification of culinary practices and tastes, Rabelais's literary text in effect rivals contemporary cookbooks and natural histories. Indeed, the stylistic richness of Rabelais's culinary vocabulary illustrates how culinary literature can rise from its ignoble station in the bowels of a grimy kitchen to take its place in a more ethereal realm of the culinary imagination where words take the place of things and dreams of satiation and savoury tastes can be resolved and sublimated. As such, rather than a denunciation of food and banqueting excess, as is suggested by the bulk of Rabelais criticism regarding the *Quart livre*, the Gaster episode is a celebration of the culinary, linguistic, and cultural inventiveness of Renaissance France.

Clearly by the mid-sixteenth century, culinary literature in France had obtained a critical mass, had reached a crucial threshold. As Pantagruel advises to his companions in his eponymous text, 'Allons enfans, c'est trop musé ici à la viande' (310) [Come, lads, there's too much thinking about food (220)]. Indeed, Pantagruel's words smack of prophecy. With the advent of the Wars of Religion, the rehabilitated status of food and culinary literature becomes subsumed within the ideological antinomies of Catholics and Protestants. Yet Rabelais provides a sense of calm before the storm. In the chapter immediately following the Gaster episode, Pantagruel has just awakened from a deep sleep occasioned by the reading of a book. The winds have failed, and so Pantagruel and his bored companions discuss how to pass the time. The ultimate solution is to dine together. At Pantagruel's ringing of the bell, which resonates with the bell rung at the start of Gaster's banquet, Frère Jean runs to the galley to prepare their meal. At the conclusion of the feast, boredom has been alleviated, questions have been resolved, and the never-ending voyage can continue. Rabelais thus posits cuisine and banqueting as an inoculation against the social ills to come. Food certainly can be perverted through improper use and, as such, is prone to raising the specter of gluttony. But it can also be a balm and a remedy in the context of conviviality, shared meals, and shared tastes. The literature of food has made this realisation possible.

Appendix A

Meat-day menu

I. Approchans les Gastrolatres je veids qu'ilz estoient suyviz d'un grand nombre de gros varletz chargez de corbeilles, de paniers, de balles, de potz, poches et marmites. Adoncques soubs la conduicte de Manduce, chantans ne sçay quelz Dithyrambes, Craepalocomes, Epaenons, offrirent a leur Dieu ouvrans leurs corbeilles et marmites

1. Hippocras blanc
2. avecques la tendre roustie seiche
3. Pain blanc
4. Choine
5. Carbonnades de six sortes
6. Coscotons
7. Fressures
8. Fricassees, neuf especes
9. Grasses souppes de prime
10. Souppes Lionnoises
11. Hoschepotz
12. Pain mollet
13. Pain bourgeoys
14. Cabirotades
15. Longes de veau rousty froides sinapisées de pouldre Zinziberine
16. Pastez d'assiette
17. Souppes de Levrier
18. Chous cabutz a la mouelle de boeuf
19. Salmiguondins

II. Brevaige eternel parmy, precedent le bon et friant vin blanc, suyvant vin clairet et vermeil frays, je vous diz froyd comme la glace: servy et offert en grandes tasses d'argent. Puys offroient

20. Andouilles capparassonnées de moustarde fine
21. Saulsisses
22. Langues de boeuf fumées
23. Saumates
24. Eschinées aux poys
25. Fricandeaux
26. Boudins
27. Cervelatz
28. Saulcissons
29. Jambons
30. Hures de Sangliers
31. Venaison sallée aux naveaulx
32. Hastereaux
33. Olives colymbades

III. Le tout associé de brevaige sempiternel. Puys luy enfournoient en gueule

34. Esclanches à l'aillade
35. Pastez à la saulse chaulde
36. Coustelettes de porc à l'oignonnade
37. Chappons roustiz avecques leur degout
38. Hutaudeaux
39. Becars
40. Cabirotz
41. Bischars
42. Dains
43. Lievres
44. Levraux
45. Perdris
46. Perdriaux
47. Faisans
48. Faisadeaux
49. Pans
50. Panneaux
51. Ciguoines
52. Ciguoineaux
53. Becasses
54. Becassins
55. Hortolans
56. Cocqs
57. poulles

58. et poulletz d'Inde
59. Ramiers
60. Ramerotz
61. Cochons au moust
62. Canars à la dodine
63. Merles
64. Rasles
65. Poulles d'eau
66. Tadournes
67. Aigrettes
68. Cercelles
69. Plongeons
70. Butors
71. Palles
72. Courlis
73. Gelinotes de boys
74. Foulques aux pourreaux
75. Risses
76. Chevreaulx
77. Espaulles de moutton aux cappres
78. Pieces de boeuf royalles
79. Poictrines de veau
80. Poulles boullies
81. et gras chappons au blanc manger
82. Gelinottes
83. Poulletz
84. Lappins
85. Lappereaux
86. Cailles
87. Cailleteaux
88. Pigeons
89. Pigeonneaux
90. Herons
91. Heronneaux
92. Otardes
93. Otardeaux
94. Becquefigues
95. Guynettes
96. Pluviers
97. Oyes
98. Oyzons
99. Bizetz
100. Hallebrans
101. Maulvyz

102. Flamans
103. Cignes
104. Pochecuillieres
105. Courtes
106. Grues
107. Tyransons
108. Corbigeaux
109. Francourlis
110. Tourterelles
111. Connilz
112. Porcespicz
113. Girardines

IV. *Ranffort de vinaige parmy. Puys*

114. grands Pastez de venaison
115. D' Allouettes
116. De Lirons
117. De Stamboucqs
118. De Chevreuilz
119. De Pigeons
120. De Chamoys
121. De Chappons
122. Pastez de lardons
123. Pieds de porc au sou
124. Croustes de pastez fricassées
125. Corbeaux de Chappons
126. Fromaiges
127. Pesches de Corbeil
128. Artichaulx
129. Guasteaux feueilletez
130. Cardes
131. Brides à veaux
132. Beuignetz
133. Tourtes de seize façons
134. Guauffres
135. Crespes
136. Patez de Coings
137. Caillebotes
138. Neige de Creme
139. Myrobalans confictz
140. Gelee
141. Hippocras rouge et vermeil
142. Poupelins
143. Macarons

144. Tartres vingt sortes
145. Crème
146. Confictures seiches et liquides soixante et dixhuyt especes
147. Dragée, cent couleurs
148. Jonchées
149. Mestier au sucre fin
150. Vinaige suyvoit à la queue de paour des Esquinanches
151. *Item* rousties

Appendix B

Meatless-day menu

I. D'entrée de table ilz lui offrent
    1. Caviat
    2. Boutargues
    3. Beurre frays
    4. Purées de poys
    5. Espinars
    6. Arans blanc bouffiz
    7. Arans sors
    8. Sardaines
    9. Anchoys
    10. Tonnine
    11. Caules emb'olif
    12. Saulgrenées de febves
Sallades cent diversitez
        13. de cresson
        14. de Obelon
        15. de la couille a l' evesque
        16. de response
        17. d' aureilles de Judas (c'est une forme de funges issans des vieulx Suzeaulx)
        18. de Aspergez
        19. de Chevrefeuel: tant d' aultres
    20. Saulmons sallez
    21. Anguillettes sallees
    22. Huytres en escalles

II. Là fault boyre, ou le Diable l'emporteroit. Ilz y donnent bon ordre, et n'y a faulte: Puys luy offrent

    23. Lamproyes a saulce d' Hippocras
    24. Barbeaulx
    25. Barbillons

26. Meuilles
27. Meuilletz
28. Rayes
29. Casserons
30. Esturgeons
31. Balaines
32. Macquereaulx
33. Pucelles
34. Plyes
35. Huytres frittes
36. Pectoncles
37. Languoustes
38. Espelans
39. Guourneaulx
40. Truites
41. Lavaretz
42. Guodepies
43. Poulpres
44. Limandes
45. Carreletz
46. Maigres
47. Pageaux
48. Gougeons
49. Barbues
50. Cradotz
51. Carpes
52. Brochetz
53. Palamides
54. Roussettes
55. Oursins
56. Vielles
57. Ortigues
58. Crespions
59. Gracieuxseigneurs
60. Empereurs
61. Anges de mer
62. Lampreons
63. Lancerons
64. Brochetons
65. Carpions
66. Carpeaux
67. Saulmons
68. Saulmonneaux
69. Daulphins
70. Porcilles

71. Turbotz
72. Pocheteau
73. Soles
74. Poles
75. Moules
76. Homars
77. Chevrettes
78. Dards
79. Ablettes
80. Tanches
81. Umbres
82. Merluz frays
83. Seiches
84. Rippes
85. Tons
86. Guoyons
87. Meusniers
88. Escrevisses
89.Palourdes
90. Liguombeaulx
91. Chatouilles
92. Congres
93. Oyes
94. Lubines
95. Aloses
96. Murenes
97. Umbrettes
98. Darceaux
99. Anguilles
100. Anguillettes
101. Tortues
102. Serpens, *id est*, Anguilles de boys.
103. Dorades
104. Poullardes
105. Perches
106. Realz
107. Loches
108. Cancres
109. Escargotz
110. Grenoilles

III. Ces viandes devorées s'il ne beuvoit, la Mort l'attendoit à deux pas pres. L'on y pourvoyoit tresbien. Puys luy estoient sacrifiez

111. Merluz sallez
112. Stocficz

113. Oeufz fritz
114. perduz
115. suffocquez
116. estuvez
117. trainnez par les cendres
118. jectez par la cheminee
119. barbouillez
120. gouildronnez, et cet.
121. Moulues
122. Papillons
123. Adotz
124. Lancerons marinez

IV. Pour les quelz cuyre et digerer facillement, vinaige estoit multiplié. Sus la fin offroient

125. Ris
126. Mil
127. Gruau
128. Beurre d'Amendes
129. Neige de beurre
130. Pistaces
131. Fisticques
132. Figues
133. Raisins
134. Escherviz
135. Millorque
136. Fromentee
137. Pruneaulx
138. Dactyles
139. Noix
140. Noizilles
141. Pasquenades
142. Artichaulx

Perennité d'abrevement parmy

Works Cited

Bakhtin, M. M. 1984. *Rabelais and his world*. Trans. Helene Iswolsky. Bloomington. Indiana University Press.

Belon, Pierre. 1555a. *L'histoire de la nature des oyseaux: avec leurs descriptions, & naïfs portraicts retirez du naturel*. Paris. G. Cauellat.

———. 1555b. *La Nature et diversité des poissons*. Paris. Charles Estienne.

————. 1997. *L'histoire de la nature des oyseaux*. Ed. Philippe Glardon. Geneva. Droz.

Berry, Alice Fiola. 2000. *The Charm of Catastrophe: A Study of Rabelais's Quart livre*. Chapel Hill. University of North Carolina Press.

Bowen, Barbara C. 1998. *Enter Rabelais, Laughing*. Nashville, TN. Vanderbilt University Press.

Brereton, Georgine E., and Janet M. Ferrier, eds. 1981. *Le menagier de Paris*. Oxford. Clarendon Press.

Bruyérin-Champier, Jean. 1560. *De re cibaria*. Lyon. Honoratum.

————. 1998. *L'alimentation de tous les peuples et de tous les temps jusqu'au XVIe siècle*. Trans. Sigurd Amundsen. Paris. Intermédiaire des Chercheurs et Curieux.

Cave, Terence. 1979. *The Cornucopian Text: Problems of Writing in the French Renaissance*. Oxford. Oxford University Press.

Cloulas, Ivan. 1985. *Henri II*. Paris. Fayard.

Cotgrave, Randle. 1611. *A Dictionarie of the French and English Tongues*. London. Adam Islip.

Demerson, Guy, and Christiane Lauvergnat-Gagnière, eds. 1982. *Le disciple de Pantagruel: les navigations de Panurge*. Société des textes français modernes 175. Paris. Nizet.

Le disciple de Pantagruel: les navigations de Panurge. 1982. Edited by Guy Demerson and Christiane Lauvergnat-Gagnière. Société des textes français modernes; 175. Paris. Nizet.

Du manuscrit à la table: Essais sur la cuisine au Moyen Age et répertoire des manuscrits médiévaux contenant des recettes culinaires. 1992. Edited by Carole Lambert. Paris, Montreal. Les Presses de l'Université de Montréal and Champion-Slatkine.

Duval, Edwin M. 1988. 'La Messe, la cène, et le voyage sans fin du *Quart livre*'. *Etudes rabelaisiennes*. 21. 131–41.

La Fleur de tout cuysine. c.1543–47. Paris. [Pierre Sergent].

Glauser, Alfred. 1966. *Rabelais créateur*. Paris. Nizet.

Gray, Floyd. 1974. *Rabelais et l'écriture*. Paris. Nizet.

Histoire de l'alimentation. 1996. Edited by Jean-Louis Flandrin and Massimo Montanari. Paris. Fayard.

Hyman, Philip, and Mary Hyman. 1992. 'Les livres de cuisine et le commerce des recettes en France aux XVe et XVIe siècles'. In *Du manuscrit à la table*. Ed. Carole Lambert. 59–68.

————. 1996. 'Imprimer la cuisine: les livres de cuisine en France entre le XVe et le XIXe siècle'. In *Histoire de l'alimentation*. Ed. Jean-Louis Flandrin and Massimo Montanari. 643–55.

————. 2001. 'Les livres de cuisine imprimés en France: Du règne de Charles VIII à la fin de l'Ancien régime'. In *Livres en bouches: Cinq siècles d'art culinaire français*. 55–75.

Jeanneret, Michel. 1987. *Des mets et des mots: banquets et propos de table à la Renaissance*. Paris. J. Corti.

Kinser, Sam. 1990. *Rabelais's Carnival: Text, Context, Metatext*. Berkeley. University of California Press.

Lestringant, Frank. 1993a. *Ecrire le monde à la Renaissance: quinze études sur Rabelais, Postel, Bodin et la littérature géographique*. Caen. Paradigme.

———. 1993b. 'L'insulaire de Rabelais, ou la fiction en archipel pour une lecture topographique du "Quart livre"'. In Frank Lestringant, *Ecrire le monde à la Renaissance*. 159–85.

———. 2002. *Le livre des îles: Atlas et récit insulaires de la Genèse à Jules Verne*. Geneva.

Livre de Cuysine. c.1539–40. Paris. [Pierre Sergent].

Livre fort excellent de cuysine. 1542. Lyon. Olivier Arnoullet.

Livres en bouches: Cinq siècles d'art culinaire français. 2001. Paris. Hermann and the Bibliothèque nationale de France.

Petit traicte. c.1536–38. Paris. [Pierre Sergent].

Pichon, Jérôme, ed. 1846. *Le Ménagier de Paris: Traité de morale et d'économie domestique composé vers 1393 par un bourgeois Parisien*. Paris. Société des bibliophiles françois.

Platina. 1505. *Platine en francoys*. Trans. Desdier Christol. Lyon. François Fradin.

———. 1998. *On Right Pleasure and Good Health*. Ed. and trans. Mary Ella Milham. Tempe, AZ. Medieval & Renaissance Texts & Studies.

Rabelais, François. 1991. *The Complete Works of François Rabelais*. Trans. Donald M. Frame. Berkeley. University of California Press.

———. 1994. *Oeuvres complètes*. Edited by Mireille Huchon. Paris. Gallimard.

Renner, Bernd. 2007a. *Difficile est saturam non scribere: l'herméneutique de la satire rabelaisienne*. Geneva. Droz.

———. 2007b. 'From the "Bien Yvres" to Messere Gaster: The Syncretism of Rabelaisian Banquets'. In *At the Table: Metaphorical and Material Cultures of Food in Medieval and Early Modern Europe*. Edited by Timothy J. Tomasik and Juliann M. Vitullo. Turnhout, Belgium. Brepols. 167–85.

Rigolot, Francois. 1972. *Les langages de Rabelais*. Geneva. Droz.

Rondelet, Guillaume. 1558. *L'Histoire entière des poissons*. Lyon. Mace Bonhomme.

Sainéan, Lazare. 1921. *L'histoire naturelle et les branches connexes dans l'oeuvre de Rabelais*. Paris. Champion.

———. 1922. *La langue de Rabelais*. Paris. Anciennes maisons Thorin et Fontemoing.

Scully, Terence, ed. 1988. *The Viandier of Taillevent: An Edition of all Extant Manuscripts*. Ottawa. University of Ottawa Press.

Taillevent. [1892]. *Le Viandier de Guillaume Tirel dit Taillevent*. Ed. Jérôme Pichon and Georges Vicaire. Luzarches. Daniel Morcrette. First published 1486.

Tomasik, Timothy J. 2003. *Textual Tastes: The Invention of Culinary Literature in Early Modern France*. Doctoral dissertation. Harvard University.

Vicaire, Georges. 1890. *Bibliographie gastronomique*. Paris. P. Rouquette.

PART 2
Early Modern Cookbooks and Recipes

Chapter 3
Recipes for Knowledge:
Maker's Knowledge Traditions,
Paracelsian Recipes, and the
Invention of the Cookbook, 1600–1660

Elizabeth Spiller

Julia Child's *Mastering the Art of French Cooking* and *The Joy of Cooking*, James Beard's *James Beard's American Cookery*, Elizabeth David's *An Omelette and a Glass of Wine*, Rick Bayless's *Rick Bayless's Mexican Kitchen*, or, further back, Fannie Farmer's *Boston Cooking-School Cookbook*. In both our own experiences and the memories that we encounter indirectly through the well-used cookbooks that are preserved in the Schlesinger and other libraries, recipe books are integral to the cultural history of food. In the Anglo-American tradition, recognisably modern versions of the recipe-book first appeared in the late seventeenth century. Recent scholarly work on the cultural history of food in the Renaissance has largely focused on the importance of Galenic humoralism and, with that, on the dietary.[1] The English cookbook of the late Renaissance did not, however, develop out of those Galenic traditions so much as in opposition to them. Indeed, the historic emergence of the modern cookbook depended on three key factors: print culture, a philosophical commitment to detailed measurement (recipes, rather than 'receipts'), and the emergence of food as a category that could be thought of as fundamentally distinct from health (cookbooks, rather than dietaries). Any history of this sort is necessarily complex and multiple in ways that tend to escape attempts to create a single narrative. Here, though, I would like to focus on an event that, while understood to be significant in the history of medicine, has not seemed important in the history of food. In 1618, the Royal College of Physicians of London published a medical remedy dispensatory, the *Pharmacopoea Londinensis*. The history and impact of this volume provides a way of understanding how print culture, measurement standards, and food categories were shifting in early seventeenth-century England. Galenism integrated well into the humanism that dominated much of early modern culture. Michael Schoenfeldt has argued that Galenic accounts of the body 'describe not so much the actual workings of the body as the

---

[1]   For a comprehensive history of the dietary, see Albala. On the impact that dietaries had on the thought and experience of the period, see Schoenfeldt, Paster, Sawday, Fitzpatrick, and Appelbaum.

experience of the body' (Schoenfeldt, 3). As Schoenfeldt and others have made clear, Galenism provided a way to describe and understand emotions and feelings within the context of the physical body. Recipe books (books of secrets, chemical remedy books, and ultimately cookbooks), by contrast, were not the products of Galenic humanism; these texts instead come out of separate mechanical, artisinal, and medical traditions that were committed to an understanding of what Antonio Pérez-Ramos has called 'maker's knowledge' in which knowing how to make something was understood to be a valid and powerful form of knowledge (Pérez-Ramos, 48–62). My larger goal in this essay is thus to trace in the history of such recipe books one part of an alternative strand of Renaissance attitudes towards the body, one which, as Pamela Smith argues, saw cognition as embodied, with the body as a site and source not of feeling but of knowledge (Smith, 9).

I take as my point of departure the *Pharmacopoea Londinensis*, which was initially published in 1618 under the auspices of the Royal College of Physicians and served, by royal decree, as the official text regulating the compounding of both Galenic and Paracelsian medicines through to at least 1649. The influential Paracelsian physician, Theodore de Mayerne, who served as James's personal physician and who had joined the Royal College of Physicians two years earlier, wrote the preface and had a significant influence on its contents and organisation. I end with a second recipe book also attributed, but in this case probably spuriously, to Mayerne: *Archimagirus Anglo-Gallicus* (1658), a small volume of strictly culinary recipes purported to have been 'copied from a choice Manuscript of Sir Theodore Mayerne, Knight, Physician to the late K. Charles' (Mayerne, title page). The iconic transformation of the king's physician into a culinary chef, an 'archimagirus', is part of a larger epistemological shift in the meaning of physic and food that enables the migration of recipes from the books of secrets that were associated with the mechanical arts tradition into recipe collections that were devoted specifically and distinctively to cooking. Looking at printed recipe books published before and after 1618, we can see the ways in which English interest in Paracelsian iatrochemistry, which featured strongly in the *Pharmacopoea Londinensis*, contributed indirectly to an overlooked reclassification of the status of food by largely removing it from the category of physic under which it had been in traditional Galenic models of the body. Paracelsianism, although never dominant as a medical system, nonetheless brought with it an emphasis on accurate measurement. Measurement was not generally consistent with Galenism, but it was necessary to the shift from recipes that relied on largely Aristotelian understandings of experience (those in the maker's knowledge tradition, which emphasised what happens all or most of the time) to recipes that followed post-Baconian ones (what happened at a particular instance). The modern form of the 'cookbook' that supplants the earlier 'books of secrets' by the middle of the seventeenth century emerges out of this reclassification of these earlier knowledge traditions surrounding food and physic.

On 26 April 1618, King James issued a royal proclamation that designated the *Pharmacopoea Londinensis*, a volume of medicinal recipes that the College of Physicians was due to publish later that year, as the country's official medical dispensatory. In this decree, James commanded that no apothecary should

> compound or make any medicine or medicinal receipt, or prescription, or distill any oyle, or waters, or other extractions, that are or shall bee in the said *Pharmacopoea Londinensis* mentioned and named after the ways or meanes prescribed or directed, by any other bookes or dispensatories whatsoever, but after the onely manner and forme, that is or shall be directed, prescribed and set downe by the sayd booke, and according to the weights and measures, that are or shall bee therein limited, and not otherwise. (James I 1618, n.p.)

James presented the *Pharmacopoea Londinensis* and the standardisation of medical practice that it represented as an important attempt to prevent 'the great danger' that variously or improperly compounded medicines might have on the 'lives and health' of his subjects.

Considered from the perspective of the social history of medicine, the 1618 Proclamation is an important landmark in the professionalisation of the practice of apothecary in England. The Worshipful Society of Apothecaries had been founded by royal charter the previous year, on 6 December 1617. Apothecaries had originally been members of one of the great livery companies of London, the Grocer's Company, and this affiliation came about because the Grocers dealt in the importing of drugs, spices, and chemicals used in medicinal compounds. Although apothecaries formed a distinct group within the Company, they nonetheless wanted to establish an independent company and were strongly supported by Gideon de Laune, Theodore de Mayerne, Henry Atkins, and other influential physicians and apothecaries connected either to the London College of Physicians or to James' court (Wall et al., 8–22; Clark. 218–32). The Society's existence depended on the transformation of what could be seen, depending on one's perspective, as a mercantile practice or mechanical art into a distinctly professional discipline. Much like the regulation of barber surgeons, the founding of the Society was intended to curtail the practice of unlicensed empirics; like attempts by the Chamberlen family to redefine midwifery, the emergence of the Society also contributed to a re-gendering of physic – once largely the responsibility of women in the private sphere – as a public domain over which men now had control.[2] The *Pharmacopoea* was integral to the mission of the Society, and, indeed, interest in having a dispensatory may have been important in consolidating interest in establishing the Society itself: the College of Physicians first expressed interest in the possibility of establishing a *liber antidotarius* as early as 1585 (Clark 158, 161; Debus 1977, 182–6). The first draft for the Society's charter (1614) also specified that the group would establish such a volume, and, when the king issued a further order that dealt with the Society of Apothecaries two years later, he again emphasised the importance of the *Pharmacopoea Londinensis*, now 'the second time renewed, corrected, and imprinted', and reaffirmed his command

---

[2]   On the Chamberlen family's attempt to incorporate midwives, see Wilson 32, 53–7.

that this volume be adhered to as part of his continuing support for the Society of Apothecaries (Wall et al., 13; James I, 1620, n.p). Within these contexts, King James's 1618 proclamation marked an important moment in the changing medical practices of Stuart England.

The 1618 proclamation in which James set out his 'express Will and Pleasure' was addressed to 'all Apothecaries of this Realme' and was intended to control the use, sale, and circulation of drugs and medicines within London. As such, James's orders regarding the *Pharmacopoea Londinensis* were part of a larger effort on the part of the crown to regulate domestic and foreign trade in spices, foodstuffs, and other market commodities. James passed a steady stream of proclamations that set restrictions on such things as making wheat or corn starch (because of dearth in grain crops) (1606), exporting uncured leather (1608), importing pepper (1609), importing felt or exporting yarn (that would make such felt) (1614), or 'garbling' (separating) spices (1622). In the same vein, James also worked to carry out Elizabeth's initiatives for establishing credible, standardized weights and measures. In 1567, Elizabeth had established a committee to update the standards for weights and measures that had been set by Henry VII in the 1490s but that had fallen into misuse. After the committee completed its work in 1601, first Elizabeth and then James passed a series of proclamations that called for an end to 'all differences and deceipts of measure' (Elizabeth I, n.p.).[3] Like these other proclamations, the 1618 order is, in part, a trade document. Furthermore, as we shall see, both the king's order and the *Pharmacopoea Londinensis* itself strongly emphasised the importance of accurate weights and measures as central to the creation of a national medical dispensatory. The new troy weights that were being sent around the country would prevent 'differences and deceipts of measure' for consumers at the market or inn; the *Pharmacopoea* would likewise ensure 'true weights and measures' for patients.

Perhaps surprisingly, given these affiliations, James's more general proclamations on weights and measures were not directed at apothecaries. In a 1619 proclamation concerning weights and measures, the king emphasised the need to exert control over weights and measures particularly for those things which involved 'the sustenance or use of mans body' (James I 1619, n.p.). James specified that these regulations should apply to, among others, millers, bakers, vinters, inn-keepers, cooks, fishmongers, grocers, and any others 'having or using weights and measures'. Despite the strong language in the 1618 proclamation about the need for true weights and measures in medicine and the obvious sense in which medicine, more than perhaps any other trade, dealt in substances for the 'use of mans body', apothecaries are notably not included on this list. It may be that the *Pharmacopoea Londinensis* was understood to have already, in the previous year, successfully addressed the abuses in physic. My sense, though, is that the apothecaries have been left off this list for a more interesting reason: in the mind of James and his ministers, apothecaries were in a substantial way no longer part of

---

[3]   See also, James I 1603, n.p.; James I 1619, n.p.

the grocer's company. For James, the affiliation between the College of Physicians and the Apothecaries changed their status ('and in that respect differed from the generall case of other Companies', as he would declare the following year), and the apothecaries themselves pursued a distinct legal status on the grounds that 'theire Arte' was 'not Mechanick, but Liberall' (James I 1620, n.p.).[4] Such a shift involves changing professional identities and fluctuating disciplinary boundaries. Perhaps more important, these new distinctions also point to a more fundamental category shift. Under the Galenic system, food and physic were integral to one another; indeed, whether a particular substance should be regarded as a form of sustenance or a type of medicine could depend on whether one was sick or healthy. With the Paracelsian assumptions that were being integrated into English medicine and culture, however, food and medicine were increasingly two quite different things, and James's attitude toward the apothecaries reflects this shift.

The implications of this category shift become more apparent when the *Pharmacopoea Londinensis* and its status as an official dispensatory are considered not just as medical events but as textual ones. That is, the publication of an official dispensatory may tell us about medical history, but it also part of a story about early modern print culture. With the 1618 Proclamation, the state was interested in promoting certain forms of medical practice, and it crucially sought to do so by tying those practices to a particular text. The binding of the text to the law was indeed quite literal: the first (May 1618) issue of the *Pharmacopoea* was set by the printers to include space for a copy of the Proclamation to be printed in the volume itself, and the summaries of the Proclamation continued to be printed in the front matter of new editions of the text long after the end of James' reign.[5] As this integration of the Proclamation into the published volume made clear, both buying and using this book became a way to follow the law. James' command thus makes the text of the *Pharmacopoea* a kind of prescription for English physic: 'We therefore desirous in all things to provide for the common good of Our Subjects, and *intending to settle and establish the generall use of the said booke in the Realme of England,* so laborously and exactly composed by the said College' (my emphasis). This emphasis on the need to 'settle and establish' a particular text as a national standard suggestively aligns the 1618 *Pharmacopoea* with two other texts that James was also committed to seeing established on a national basis: the King James Bible and the Book of Common Prayer (James I 1604, n.p.). This sense that the *Pharmacopoea* should have a kind of scriptural status was one that Mayerne encouraged in his preface to the volume, while Nicholas Culpeper would later mock this quasi-religious standing of the volume in his 1649 translation of

---

[4]   The Society's arguments for distinguishing themselves from mechanical artists arose in debates over their rank and rating among the great livery companies and are cited from Wall et al., 29.

[5]   Some of the remaining copies of the May issue have the Proclamation; others have simply a blank, suggesting that there may have been a strong demand for the volume when it was published. See Urdang, 306.

the dispensatory. Attacking both priests and physicians ('one deceives men in matters belonging to the Souls, the other in matters belonging to their Bodies'), Culpeper clearly regarded the Latin dispensatory as a kind of medical Vulgate, which prevented readers, especially women, from the knowledge that his English translation sought to make available to them (Culpeper, A1r).

Like the vernacular Bible, the *Pharmacopoea Londinensis* was, in both its form and content, a distinctive product of early modern print culture. As George Clark commented in his discussion of the spread of new pharmaceutical standards across Europe, 'the invention of printing made it possible to insist on a real uniformity of pharmaceutical standards' (Clark, 158). The impact that the printing press had on the dissemination of knowledge in early modern Europe was of course considerable (Eisenstein, 43–162, 520–74). Printing changed both what could be known and who could know it. Although printing changed many fields, it had a particularly strong impact, at the level of both form and content, on a variety of texts that pursued a connection between art, use, and knowledge that was antithetical to the Aristotelianism that had dominated learning in the age of the manuscript. These texts included practical handbooks in various mechanical arts, manuals, and recipe books. As William Eamon makes clear, such handbooks were the intellectual descendants of the pseudo-Aristotelian *Secretum Secretorum*, purportedly a collection of letters from Aristotle to Alexander the Great (Eamon, 3–12, 38–90, 93–105). Whereas Aristotle had insisted that art and nature had no epistemological connection with one another ('Art is concerned neither with things that are, or come into being, by necessity, nor with things that do so in accordance with nature' [Aristotle, 1140a 13ff]), the *Secretum Secretorum* seemed to promise readers that art and nature were not distinct, and that art indeed provided a means to gain knowledge from and power over nature.

Carla Mazzio and Bradin Cormack have suggested that early printed books were distinctive in being 'primarily understood as instrumental'. Texts were both tools for doing things and, in that, ways of knowing them. Mazzio and Cormack astutely conclude that 'to use a book is to engage with it as a set of forms and as a condition of thought. In this sense, the history of book use and the history of theoretical speculation are entwined' (Mazzio and Cormack, 4). The connection between how books were used and how such use was connected to the theories of knowledge embedded within those texts is particularly acute in the case of recipe books. Pushing against Aristotelian scholasticism, the books of secrets that followed from the *Secretum Secretorum* assumed that nature could be controlled by art. These texts did not offer their readers philosophy or science. Instead, they provided precisely the kind of instrumental knowledge that was associated with what, for Aristotle, had been two lesser kinds of wisdom: making (poesis) and doing (praxis).[6] The texts, part of the larger maker's knowledge tradition, were

---

[6]   For accounts that emphasize different aspects of this turn against Aristotelianism in the mechanical arts, see, among others, Eamon; Turner, 46–54; Zilsel 1941; Zilsel 1942; Rossi.

thus committed to the assumption that knowledge arises out of the arts of the hand, created in the mind but also shaped by and through the body.

Recipes first appear, in print sources, primarily in the books of secrets. In this context, recipes are thus connected to philosophical interest in using art to control nature. In England, probably the first of these books to have a substantial readership was William Ward's translation of *The Secretes of the Reverende Maister Alexis of Piedmont*, which was published in 1558 and was followed by three additional parts, in almost a dozen editions, before a composite edition was published in 1595. Other popular books of secrets were associated with English authors and included: *The boke of Secrets of Albertus Magnus* (1560); John Partridge's *Treasurie of Commodious Conceits, & Hidden Secrets* (1572); and Hugh Plat's *The Jewell House of Art and Nature* (1594).[7] The authors of these volumes promised, as Plat expressed it, 'to disclose and manifest, even those secret and hidden magisteries, both of art and nature' (Plat A2r). For Plat, art was neither separate from nor secondary to nature: 'nature', he insisted, 'may be knowne to bee so cunning an artist, as that she hath not made any thing in vaine, the wittee of man hath also founde out some good use this way' (Plat 49). The books of secrets tended to be multi-part volumes made up of a number of different books, each concerned with what seem to us to be quite different kinds of inventions, experiments, and recipes. Plat's *Jewell House*, for instance, contains separate books on experiments, husbandry, chemical distillery, and moulding, while *The boke of Secrets* begins with sections on the virtues of herbs, stones, and animals. Partridge's *Treasurie* includes more culinary material, but even here, much of the book is devoted to 'kitchen physic', with recipes for oils, extracts, salves, and other substances that would be used for medicinal purposes. The different mechanical arts that come together in such volumes – instructions for distilling, cryptography, medicinal salves, dyeing, and cooking – were allied with one another to the extent that they were understood to be 'arts of the hand' and, equally important, instances of the knowledge that such arts could produce.

Cooking is notably not a distinct category within these volumes. Food meant something quite different to recipe book authors such as Hugh Plat or John Partridge than it did to dietary writers such as Thomas Cogan and William Bullein. In the dietaries, food was theoretically understood to be one of the six non-naturals that gave men a way to control the body and its passions, and some dietaries would thus describe the virtues associated with different foods and make recommendations about the kinds of foods that different kinds of people should eat. In practice, however, dietaries did not typically include recipes, which were not inherently consistent with Galenic assumptions about the individuality of both temperament and treatment. In Partridge's *Treasurie,* for instance, the culinary recipes at the start of the book are simply presented ('To bake chickens'), but the medicinal recipes include both instructions ('To make Conserve of Roses, or Other

---

7   For accounts of the books of secrets in the English tradition, see Spiller, xii–xvi; Wall, 42–53; Kavey.

Flowers') and commentary about their efficacy ('The vertue of the conserve of Roses') that come out of a Galenic tradition (Partridge, C1r). The dietaries tended to refer to cooking itself largely in metaphoric terms, as a way to describe how the human body worked. From this perspective, concocting, distilling, and cooking all had their counterparts within the human digestive process. In the recipe books, by contrast, the emphasis is on the control of nature, not that of man. Man controls; he is not that which is controlled. For someone like Platt, cooking is a mechanical art that is significant to the extent that it can transform nature and, thus, create something perhaps more real than nature itself.

Although cooking is initially subordinate to physic within the books of secrets, the shift away from Galenic models of the body tended to create an intellectual space for cooking as a category in its own right. This category shift is apparent in the publication histories of these volumes. Books of secrets were introduced to English readers in the middle of the sixteenth century and were at the height of their popularity in the last quarter of the century. The first wave of books of secrets, which included the volumes attributed to Alexis of Piedmont and Albertus Magnus, were initially published in the 1550s and 1560s. These volumes went through multiple editions and were usually printed by more than one printer. While additional materials and even sequels were added in the later editions, these volumes were fairly consistent in combining the various mechanical arts into a single philosophical structure and narrative form. The second wave of publications includes those works published from about 1575 to about 1600, and representative titles here would include: John Partridge's *The Treasurie of Commodious Conceits* (1573) and *The Widowes Treasure* (1586, 2nd ed.), the composite *The Treasurie of Hidden Secrets* (1596), Thomas Dawson's *The Good Huswifes Jewell* (1596) and his *Booke of cookerie* (1620), Hugh Plat's *The Jewell House of Art and Nature* (1594) and his *Delightes for Ladies* (1602), and the anonymous *A Closet for Ladies and Gentlewomen* (1608), which was often bound with Plat's *Delightes*. In the works from this group, cooking is still associated, at a philosophical level, with the mechanical arts and the books of secrets, but that connection appears in a new textual format. Plat's *Jewell House* is a typical book of secrets; his later *Delightes for Ladies* focuses almost entirely on confectionary recipes. Partridge's *Treasurie of Commodious Conceits* (1573) is likewise a typical compendium of recipes in kitchen physic, husbandry, and cookery; 20 years later, Partridge's volume was repackaged into a composite volume, *The Treasurie of Hidden Secrets* (1596), and updated by the addition of a cookery book, *A Good huswives handmaid for the kitchen*. The addition of cooking as a more fully distinguished supplement to what had been multi-use volumes involves a shift in marketing and publication practices, and one that suggests that cooking is becoming a category in its own right.

Recipes also appear prominently in a second category of printed works from this period, that of chemical remedy books. These manuals were written by and for surgeons and apothecaries, as well as for householders who may have sought information for making household medicines. These recipe books were printed versions of stillroom books, and they were devoted to the practice of 'kitchen physic'. Among the earliest of the volumes in this category were two widely influential translations of Conrad Gesner's medical works, *The Treasure of Euonymus* (1559) and its continuation *The Newe Jewell of Health* (1576). Gesner's remedies were largely chemical and alchemical. Giving a definition of distillation at the start of the first volume, Gesner makes this focus clear: his goal is to show how complex medicinal compounds can be created 'out of simple medicines by the strengthe of fire' (Gesner Air). Although Gesner himself was not a supporter of Paracelsus, Allen Debus argues that his remedy books promoted chemical medicine in ways that ultimately worked to make Paracelsian iatrochemistry acceptable to English readers (Debus 1965, 52–3). Paracelsian and other chemical remedies are prominent in later remedy books such as Leonardo Fioravanti's *A Joyful Jewell* (1579), which was translated by the apothecary John Hester, Thomas Vicary's *The English Mans Treasure* (1586?), John Banister's *An Antidotarie Chyrurgical* (1589), and Gesner's *The Practise of New and Old Physicke* (1599). The chemical remedy books have strong intellectual affiliations with the books of secrets. Paracelsian medicine was associated closely with the mechanical arts, while alchemy as a whole was tied to the belief that human art provided the basis for the transformation of nature and the creation of knowledge. Despite their different audiences, these volumes thus often use a language that is close to that in the books of secrets. *The Treasure*, for instance, promises to reveal the 'wonderful hid secrets of nature' (Gesner, title page).

The recipes in the remedy books differ conceptually from those in the books of secrets. John Banister warns his readers that many of his recipes are 'bitter, biting, & painful, serving wher neither ease, nor delight of taste, but recoveries of health requireth to be cared for' (Banister, *2v). In saying this, Banister is in part repeating a basic tenet of Galenic medicine: food tastes good and medicine tastes bad because food is like the healthy body that it nourishes and so is absorbed by it, while medicine is unlike the sick body that it heals and so assimilates that body to itself (Siraisi, 121). Although Banister begins with this Galenic framework, his recipes nonetheless are structured in ways that follow Paracelsian assumptions. Culinary recipes from this period – recipes that are indeed concerned with 'delight of taste' – tend to provide fairly imprecise measurements. Partridge, whose recipes in *The Treasurie of Commodious Conceits* are of a comparatively high standard, provides more and less quantifiable measurements: for red sealing wax, for instance, he recommends 3 ounces of clear turpentine, but specifies 4 ounces in winter. In Partridge's culinary recipes, quantity itself is a unit of measurement: different recipes specify, in slightly different modulations, 'a quantity of butter', 'a good quantity of butter', and 'a good quantity of sugar and cream with sufficient salt' (Partridge, D2r, F1r). Partridge's attitude toward measurement in part reflects a sense that cooking is an art, variable in practice and hard to convey in words. Equally importantly, however, this sense that both quantities and results will differ also reflects the infinite variability that was understood to characterise the humoral body: in this context, what nourishes and thus what 'tastes' good are as different as each individual's humoral complexion. Chemical remedy books like Banister's bring an attention to the standardisation of remedies and precision of measurement that accord with their understanding of Paracelsian physic. Banister thus calls attention to the need for a uniformity that inheres in the medicine not in the patient: each of his recipes begins with a list of ingredients and measurements, given in Latin and set in an italic font, clearly set off from the instructions themselves, which are English, in a blackletter typeface.

The chemical remedy books are also affiliated with the books of secrets in their relationship to print culture. The authors and printers of these volumes consistently stress the importance of making knowledge accessible in English to those who read. The printer John Daye, who is most well known for his printing of religious texts and translations, thus includes a letter in his anonymous edition of *The Treasure of Euonymus* in which he explains his decision to commission a translation of this work. Noting that people often die when medicines are improperly prepared, Daye explains that he 'caused this precious treasure to be translated into oure usuall, and native language, that like as all men are subjected to sickness so likewise all men may by this occasion learne the way to helth' (Gesner, †iir). The barber surgeons from St. Bartholomew's Hospital who 'revived, corrected, and published' Thomas Vicary's handbook on anatomy and chemical physic likewise emphasise that they are making Vicary's work available in English to remedy the need, among apprentices and surgeons, for accessible texts: 'many good and learned men', they note, 'in these our daies, do cease to publish abroad in the English tongue their works and travelles' (Vicary A4r–A4v). In a dedicatory letter to John Banister's *Antidotarie Chyrurgicall* (1589), William Goodrus alludes to the resistance faced by those who translated and disseminated closely held medical secrets. For Goodrus, the act of publishing was likely to be dangerous to one's health: addressing Banister, he writes that he wishes

> at the publishing of your *Antidotarie*, to write as an *Antidote* unto your selfe: desiring, that according to the nature of such medicines, which both expel poysons alreadies received, and also keepe and preserve the heart, against all new infections; so this may both ridde you of the present perplexities, and likewise defend you from future, against all your enemies. (Banister 5)

The translators and authors of English dietaries included humanists like Thomas Elyot and physicians like William Bullein; the translators and authors of the remedy books, who were usually surgeons, apothecaries, and technical translators working in other vernacular languages, came from a different social class and had different intellectual assumptions. As Eamon notes more generally, 'when apothecaries, potters, sailors, distillers, and midwives got into print along with scholars, humanists, and clerics, the Republic of Letters was permanently changed' (Eamon, 94). The knowledge that these texts sought to convey and create in readers crucially occurs both in the vernacular and in print.

The recipes that appear in the books of secrets and the medical remedy books provide some sense of the intellectual and cultural background against which the *Pharmacopoea Londinensis* was conceived. Print culture provided the technology that made possible the standardisation of medical practice that the *Pharmacopoea Londinensis* was interested in achieving. Printing, itself a key product of innovation in the mechanical arts, was connected both philosophically and culturally to the maker's knowledge tradition. At the same time, though, the *Pharmacopoea Londinensis* was a strong reaction against the new knowledge, and the new categories for knowledge, that print culture seemed to be stimulating. As a text, the *Pharmacopoea Londinensis* was intended to prevent the dissemination of knowledge and practice at least as much as it was designed to encourage it. The *Pharmacopoea* was, for both the College of Physicians and the king himself, a partial solution to a textual problem created by the possibilities of print culture. Observing that the 'custom of publishing private collections of medicinal recipes had been noted with alarm' in the Elizabethan period, Debus reports that 'there was a noticeable slackening of interest in the private collections of remedies after 1618' (Debus 1965, 149, 154). The publication of the *Pharmacopoea Londinensis* successfully challenged the publication of unauthorised recipe books, deriving from both the books of secrets and chemical physic. From 1618 to 1649, almost no new recipe collections of any kind appeared in print. *The Chyrugians Closet* (1630), a posthumously published collection of Paracelsian remedies from the physician Thomas Bonham, and the anonymous *Ladies Cabinet Opened* (1639) are among the few exceptions. This concern about remedy books is itself part of what Lynette Hunter has identified as a much wider reaction in the late sixteenth and early seventeenth centuries against those who were printing, selling, and buying books connected to the maker's knowledge traditions (Hunter, 99–100).

Enormously influential and repeatedly reprinted, the *Pharmacopoea* largely put an end to the printed recipe books that had dominated late sixteenth- and early seventeenth-century publishing. It is not until about 1650 that English printers again begin publishing recipe books in any kind of numbers, when we see a sudden wave of recipe books which included such works as Elizabeth Grey's *Choice Manual*, which was published jointly with *A True Gentlewoman's Delight* (1653), W. M.'s *Queens Closet Opened* (1655), Sir Kenelm Digby's *Cure of Wounds* (1658), and Robert May's *Accomplisht Cook* (1660), among others. The appearance of these volumes has rightly been tied by food historians to the remarkable impact that new developments in French cookbooks, especially Pierre François de la Varenne's *Le Cuisinier Francois* (1651; translated as *The French Cook* [1653]), had on English food culture. Despite the attention given to Varenne's work, though, the English recipe books that are published during this period notably do not incorporate continental innovations in any significant way and should probably not be understood primarily as responses to Varenne's work. Instead, I would suggest that the publication of these new recipe books instead followed from and were in some sense made possible by Nicholas Culpeper's translation of the *Pharmacopoea* into English in 1649. The success of Culpeper's translation – which he understood to be a radical act against the controls imposed on the publication of recipe books – seems to have convinced publishers to return to the once lucrative recipe book market. Although the *Pharmacopoea* continued to be published and remained the standard work, the existence of an English translation broke one of the key restrictions against publications in this genre and so restarted the publication of recipe books.

The textual monopoly that was given to the *Pharmacopoea* largely put an end to the publication of recipe books in England for more than 30 years, but somewhat ironically, the *Pharmacopoea* itself in two important respects encouraged assumptions that were important to the form and content of recipe books that emerge in the 1650s when that monopoly is broken. Both of these changes were a consequence of the way that the *Pharmacopoea* moved away from Galenism. Containing 932 compound medicines alongside 1025 simples and with the notable inclusion of a section on 'chemical' physic, the volume promoted a move away from Galenic herbalism toward Paracelsian iatrochemistry.[8] Mayerne, who probably wrote the prefatory materials to the volume, signalled this shift at the start of the 1618 editions:

> we venerate the age-old learning of the ancients and for this reason we have
> placed their remedies at the beginning, but, on the other hand, we neither reject
> nor spurn the new subsidiary medicines of the more recent chemists and we
> have conceded to them a place and corner in the rear so that they might be
> as a servant to the dogmatic medicine, and thus they might act as auxilliaries.
> (Culpeper, B2r)

Mayerne's comments understate the importance of Paracelsianism in the *Pharmacopoea*: the shift toward Paracelsian iatrochemistry was not limited to the short section on chemical remedies. Rather, this influence makes itself more profoundly felt, first, in a category shift that allowed for the separation of food from physic, of cooking from medicine; and, second, in a methodological shift that emphasised the need for standardised measurement. In both Galenism and the maker's knowledge traditions, food and physic were integrally connected to one another. From a Galenic perspective, dietary change allowed one to correct humoral imbalances, and, in the dietaries, food was thus often the inverse to physic. In the books of secrets, culinary and medicinal recipes were both instances of arts that could transform nature and did so through the body. Recipes for confections and for salves both were part of the same context and, as we have seen, part of the same texts. The *Pharmacopoea*, by contrast, was a medical remedy book that split food from physic. The *Pharmacopoea* included many traditional Galenic recipes within its pages, but its exclusion of all culinary recipes may be a more powerful indicator of the extent to which the dispensatory broke with the traditions that dominated sixteenth-century attitudes toward the body and the human art that might sustain it. By encouraging the treatment of food and medicine as distinct substances, the *Pharmacopoea Londinensis*, itself a recipe book limited to physic, helped prepare the way for the appearance of a significantly new category of recipe books devoted to cookery that becomes dominant by the end of the century.

The other distinctive feature of the *Pharmacopoea* was its attention to recipes and instructions that follow, as Mayerne noted, 'one and the same rule'. As Peter

---

[8]   Wall et al., 28; on the influx of Paracelsian iatrochemistry into England and Mayerne's role in introducing it into the *Pharmacopoea*, see Debus 1965, 150–56; Debus 1977, 173–91; Debus 1987.

Dear, Alfred Crosby, and others have argued, the 'measure of all things' changed in early modern Europe (Dear, 1–9; Crosby 3–20; 129–39; Blank, 1–40). This attempt to regulate measurement and fix ingredients was part of a larger intellectual shift away from an Aristotelian physics that was founded on qualitative assessments (a physics that was concerned with why) toward an experimental science that was based on quantitative ones (a mathematics of how many). Mayerne's prefatory letter explains their attention to creating recipes for compounding that follow 'one and the same rule' and specify a 'certain quantity or dose':

> whereas in most Authors, some things are totally left to the judgment of the Artificer, especially in the quantity of Honey and Sugar, under these two letters, q. s. or words [so much as is sufficient] whence it comes to pass that the same medicine hath neigther the some consistence nor the same vertue, we have for the future taken away this power from the Artificer, and for this cause have take some of the most skilful Apothecaries into counsel with us, by whose help and pains we have agreed upon a certain manner of composition, and designed a certain quantity and dose, which they may not ad to not take from. (Culpeper, B1v, B2r; 'Candido Lectori', Royal College, A1r, A1v)

Under a Galenic understanding of the body, substances such as sugar and honey were understood to be medicinally subtle: like herbs and spices, sugar provided a way to 'temper' foods and medicines to bring them into fuller humoral balance.[9] The amount of sugar needed to temper something would depend in part on the food or medicine, but it would also depend more fundamentally on the humoral disposition of the patient. Adding sugar or honey to taste, in the ways that Mayerne refers to here, was not primarily understood to be a matter of individual preference. (A cultural commitment to 'taste' as a marker of individuality does not become dominant until the eighteenth century). Rather, because of the way that medicine and food either absorb or are absorbed into the body, how something tastes is connected to its medical efficacy.

Traditional humoral medicine thus resisted universal cures: under a Galenic system, the kinds of fixed recipes *Pharmacopoea* wanted to set as standards would not have been accepted as the basis for effective individual therapy. Hippocrates, for instance, asserts that 'no measure, neither number nor weight, by reference to which knowledge can be made exact, can be found except bodily feeling' (Hippocrates, *Of Ancient Medicine*; cited in Appelbaum, 53). Paracelsianism, by contrast, moved away from this systemic model and, as Debus notes, 'went to great pains to determine the correct dosage with their medicines' (Debus 1965, 34). This emphasis on standardised measurement and the setting of recipes was associated closely with the *Pharmacopoea* as a whole and with Theodore de Mayerne in particular. In *Some considerations touching the usefulnesse of experimental natural philosophy* (London, 1663), Robert Boyle includes a long appendix that dealt with the way in which the new science of chemistry was improving the preparation of medical remedies. Boyle is committed to chemical physic, but he remains

---

[9]   On the medicinal qualities attributed to sugar, see Albala, 66, 179; Mintz, 96–108.

wary of 'particular receipts' (Boyle, 399). Boyle gently mocks those physicians who believe that a single compound could provide a universal cure 'in Persons of all Ages, Sexes, and Complexions, indiscriminately' and cites 'the famous Sir Theodore Mayerne' as his example of this kind of 'Methodist' (Boyle, 401).

The need for precise and standard forms of measurement certainly becomes increasingly important in the recipe books that were published after 1618. Leonard Sowerby's *Ladies Dispensatory* (1651), for instance, includes a table of measurement equivalences as a supplement to his recipes. Aletheia Talbot's *Natura exenterata* (1655) instructs readers to distinguish differently sized handfuls for different ingredients: herbs should be measured by the full handful (marked M.) but flowers by the small handful (marked P.): 'that is to say the first must be a good handfull and the latter a little handfull' (Talbot 347 [374]). Culpeper also inserts a supplemental page on weights and measures in the prefatory materials to his translation in which he provides a series of equivalences (scruples to drams to ounces) and translations for Roman and Greek forms of measure (libra to ounce, for instance) (Culpeper, B3v). Beyond this, however, he also complains that

> besides these, the College have gotten another foolish and incertain way of measuration not here set down, viz. by handfuls and pugills, what a handfull is, is known to all, but how much it is, is known to none, but is as different as mens hands are in bigness or their fingers in length. A pugil is properly so much as you can take up with your thumb and two fingers, and is very uncertain, not only in respect of the length of the finger, but also in respect of the matter you can take up, for your mothers wit will tell you, you may take up more hay in that manner than bran. (Culpeper, B3v)

Despite the strong emphasis that the College of Physicians had placed on instituting more accurate forms of measurement, critics such as Culpeper were committed to even more profound changes. The handful and pugil – along with other measurements of the body like the yard, the foot, the ell, and the span – were less a measurement system than a form of proportional ratio in which man was the measure of all things. Paracelsianism shifted away from both the variable humoral body, with its radically individual complexions and its assumption that man existed in relation to the world as a whole, and the variable human centre to ratio measurement, with its 'foolish and uncertain form of measuration'. This shift was important to the transformation of the kinds of recipes that had prevailed in the books of secrets to those that became central to cookbooks.

One of the recipe books that appeared in this wave of publications from the 1650s was a small volume entitled *Archimagirus Anglo-Gallicus* (1658). The primary printer of the volume was Gabriel Bedell, who had recently published several editions of Lord Ruthven's *Ladies Cabinet Enlarged* (1654, 1655, 1658) and Talbot's *Natura Exenterata* (1655). As his title suggested, Bedell clearly sought to capture readers who might be interested in recent French innovations. This appeal to a desire for new forms of continental cooking is, however, largely restricted to the title page: there are a handful of recipes here that are influenced by developments in French and Italian cooking, but on the whole the recipes in the *Archimagirus Anglo-Gallicus* (beginning with meat pies and savoury dishes, seasoned with nutmeg, cinnamon, cloves and mace, and ending with quintessentially English sugar works and preserves) are resolutely English in character. Bedell's title page thus makes a second appeal to potential readers by promising that these recipes were 'copied from a choice Manuscript of Sir *Theodore Mayerne* knight, Physician to the late K. Charles' (Mayerne, title page). This appeal is more in keeping with the character of the other, aristocratic recipe books he was publishing during this period, and one that suggestively points to the influence that the *Pharmacopoea Londinensis* had on the publication of recipe books, both chemical and culinary, in seventeenth-century England.

Bedell promises his readers that these recipes are Mayerne's. In a literal sense, this claim is almost certainly not true: there is no good bibliographic or biographical reason to suppose that the recipes in this volume were Mayerne's; indeed, the recipes themselves, while traditional in some respects, probably date from the middle of the seventeenth century rather than from the late sixteenth or early seventeenth century, as one would expect if were they Mayerne's. In a more figurative sense and insofar as this volume represents both that which is excluded from the *Pharmacopoea Londinensis* and that which is the intellectual consequence of it, though, these recipes and this recipe book might well be Theodore de Mayerne's. The *Archimagirus Anglo-Gallicus* is a small volume, published comparatively inexpensively in octavo. It is a three-part volume: the first and longest section devoted to culinary recipes, the second to 'experiments' in sugar work, and the final and shortest section to recipes for preserving. The culinary recipes are mostly traditional meat pies and dishes (calf's head pie seasoned with sugar, neat's tongue, wild boar). Many of the recipes in the final section adhere to the traditions and practices that informed the work of Platt and Partridge (including one recipe that promises pancakes 'as crispe as wafers' and 'as yellow as gold') (Mayerne, 71). These features of the volume stand at odds, though, with the unsigned practice to the volume.

Praising the 'Excellency of Kitchen-Physick', the author of this dedicatory epistle suggests that this volume will give you 'the Doctour's Cooke', and so 'will teach you to keep good houses, by keeping good things in them' (Mayerne, A2v, A3v). The volume itself does not, however, contain any of the kitchen-physic here praised: indeed, the structure of the volume, in which cooking has now replaced physic, distinguishes this volume from pre-1618 recipe books. In its structure and its contents, *Archimagirus Anglo-Gallicus* offers evidence of how Maynerne's *Pharmacopoea* insisted upon the science of physic, as was its intention, and, in doing so, created a new category for cooking as an art in its own right.

Works Cited

Albala, Ken. 2002. *Eating Right in the Renaissance*. Berkeley. University of California Press.

Appelbaum, Robert. 2006. *Aguecheek's Beef, Belch's Hiccup, and other Gastronomic Interjections*. Chicago, IL. University of Chicago Press.

Aristotle. 1984. *Nicomachean Ethics*. Trans. W. D. Ross and J. O. Urmson. *The Complete Works of Aristotle*. 2 vols. Ed. Jonathan Barnes. Princeton, NJ: Bollingen Series. Princeton University Press. 1729–1867.

Banister, John. 1589. *An Antidotarie Chyrurgicall*. London. Thomas Orwin for Thomas Man.

Blank, Paula. 2006. *Shakespeare and the Mismeasure of Renaissance Man*. Ithaca. NY. Cornell University Press.

Boyle, Robert. 1663. *Some considerations touching the usefulness of experimental natural philosophy*. London. Hen[ry]. Hall for Ric[hard]. Davis.

Clark, George. 1964. *A History of the Royal College of Physicians of London*. Vol. 1. Oxford. Clarendon Press.

Crosby, Alfred W. 1997. *The Measure of Reality: Quantification in Western Europe, 1250–1600*. Cambridge. Cambridge University Press.

Culpeper, Nicholas, trans. 1649. *A Physical Directory, or a Translation of the London Dispensatory*. London.

Dear, Peter. 1985. *Discipline and Experience: The Mathematical Way in the Scientific Revolution*. Chicago, IL. University of Chicago Press.

Debus, Allen G. 1965. *The English Paracelsians*. London. Oldbourne Press.

———. 1977. *The Chemical Philosophy: Paracelsian Science and Medicine in the Sixteenth and Seventeenth Centuries*. New York. Science History Publications.

———. 1987. 'The Paracelsians and the Chemists: The Chemical Dilemma in Renaissance Medicine'. *Chemistry, Alchemy, and the New Philosophy 1550–1700*. London. Variorum Reprints. 185–99.

Eamon, William. 1994. *Science and the Secrets of Nature: Books of Secrets in Medieval and Early Modern Culture*. Princeton, NJ. Princeton University Press. 1994.

Eisenstein, Elizabeth. 1980. *The Printing Press as an Agent of Change*. Cambridge. Cambridge University Press.

Elizabeth I. 1602. 'A Proclamation for Measures'. London. Robert Barker.

Fitzpatrick, Joan. 2007. *Food in Shakespeare: Early Modern Dietaries and the Plays*. Literary and Scientific Cultures of Early Modernity. Aldershot. Ashgate.

Gesner, Conrad. 1559. *The Treasure of Euonymus*. London. John Daie.

Hunter, Lynette. 1997. 'Women and Domestic Medicine: Lady Experimenters, 1570–1620'. *Women, Science, and Medicine: Mothers and Sisters of the Royal Society*. Ed. Lynnette Hunter and Sarah Hutton. Phoenix Mill. Sutton. 89–107.

James I. 1603. 'A Proclamation for Reformation of Great Abuses in Measures'. London. Robert Barker.

———. 1604. 'Proclamation for the Authorizing and Uniformity of the Book of Common Prayer'. London. Robert Barker. 1604.

———. 1618. 'A Proclamation commanding all Apothecaries'. London. Bonham Norton and John Bill.

————.1619. 'A Proclamation for Reformation of the great abuses in Weights and Measures'. London. Bonham Norton, and John Bill.

————. 1620. 'A Proclamation for setling the Company of Apothecaries of London'. London. Bonham Norton, and John Bill.

Kavey, Allison. 2007. *Books of Secrets: Natural Philosophy in English, 1550–1600*. Chicago and Urbana. University of Illinois Press.

Mayerne, Theodore de (attributed). 1658. *Archimagirus Anglo-Gallicus*. London. Printed for G. Bedell, and T. Collins

Mazzio, Carla, and Bradin Cormack. 2005. *Book Use, Book Theory: 1500–1700*. Chicago, IL. University of Chicago Press.

Mintz, Sidney W. 1985. *Sweetness and Power: The Place of Sugar in Modern History*. New York. Viking.

Partridge, John. 1573. *The Treasurie of Commodious Conceits*. London. Richarde Jones.

Paster, Gail Kern. 1993. *The Body Embarrassed: Drama and the Disciplines of Shame in Early Modern Europe*. Ithaca, NY. Cornell University Press.

Pérez-Ramos, Antonio. 1989. *Francis Bacon's Idea of Science and the Maker's Knowledge Tradition*. Oxford. Oxford University Press.

Plat, Hugh. 1594. *The Jewell House of Art and Nature*. London. Peter Short.

Rossi, Paolo. 1970. *Philosophy, Technology, and the Arts in the Early Modern Era*. Trans. Salvator Attanasio. Ed. Benjamin Nelson. New York. Harper and Row.

Royal College of Physicians of London. 1618. *Pharmocopoea Londinensis*. London. Edwardus Griffin for Johannis Marriot.

Sawday, Jonathan. 1996. *The Body Emblazoned: Dissection and the Human Body in Renaissance Culture*. New York. Routledge.

Schoenfeldt, Michael G. 2002. *Bodies and Selves in Early Modern England: Physiology and Inwardness in Spenser, Shakespeare, Herbert, and Milton*. Cambridge. Cambridge University Press.

Siraisi, Nancy. 1990. *Medieval and Early Renaissance Medicine: Introduction to Knowledge and Practice*. Chicago, IL. University of Chicago Press.

Smith, Pamela H. 2006. *The Body of the Artisan: Art and Experience in the Scientific Revolution*. Chicago, IL. University of Chicago Press.

Spiller, Elizabeth. 2008. *Seventeenth-Century English Recipe Books: Cooking, Physic, and Chirurgery in the Works of Elizabeth Talbot Grey and Aletheia Talbot Howard*. Aldershot. Ashgate.

Talbot, Aletheia. 1655. *Natura exenterata*. London. Printed for H. Twiford.

Turner, Henry S. 2006. *The English Renaissance Stage: Geometry, Poetics, and the Practical Spatial Arts, 1580–1630*. Oxford. Oxford University Press.

Urdang, George. 1942. 'The Mystery about the First English (London) Pharmacopeia (1618)'. *Bulletin of the History of Medicine*. 12.2. 304–13.

Vicary, Thomas. 1596. *The English Mans Treasure*. London. Thomas Creede

Wall, Cecil M., et al. 1963. *A History of the Worshipful Society of Apothecaries of London, vol. 1, 1617–1815*. London. Oxford University Press.

Wall, Wendy. 2002. *Staging Domesticity: Household Work and English Identity in Early Modern Drama*. Cambridge. Cambridge University Press.

Wilson, Adrian. 1995. *The Making of Man-Midwifery: Childbirth in England, 1660–1770*. Cambridge. Harvard University Press.

Zilsel, Edgar. 1941. 'The Origins of William Gilbert's Scientific Method'. *Journal for the History of Ideas*. 2.1. 1–32.

———. 1942. 'The Sociological Roots of Science'. *The American Journal of Sociology*. 49. 544–62.

Chapter 4
Cooking as Research Methodology: Experiments in Renaissance Cuisine

Ken Albala

This essay seeks to redress a long-standing epistemological division in food scholarship. The radical separation of academic food historians from culinary historians and practitioners has had various deleterious effects. One is the tendency of academic food historians to misunderstand specific food references in historical, literary, and artistic texts, stemming from unfamiliarity with the practical conditions of historic kitchens. The other negative effect is the professional marginalization of those with technical skills whose experience is indispensible for a full appreciation of the embodied experience of our forebears and what was, for the vast majority of people, a daily activity: providing and preparing food. This essay will argue that the two disparate fields of food history and culinary history must necessarily be joined, and it will provide concrete examples of how getting one's hands dirty, so to speak, clarified what would have otherwise been inscrutable historical texts deriving from the late medieval and early modern period.

The texts in question are cookbooks, valuable for the insights they offer regarding not only domestic life, social history and gender roles but also the entire culture of food, which includes dietary and religious attitudes toward consumption and manners, as well as purely material factors such as trade networks, agriculture, and the economy. Professional historians have been analyzing cookbooks as texts for many centuries. In fact, the oldest surviving food history in the Western tradition is the *Deipnosophistae* by Athenaeus of Naucratis, who wrote in Egypt in the late second century A.D. It analyzes at great length cookbooks, such as that by Archestratus, as well as literary texts. In the eighth century, although analysis per se may not have been the impetus for making two manuscript copies of the classical cookbook attributed to Apicius, their recovery in the fifteenth century by Renaissance humanists was definitely motivated by historical concerns. Furthermore, we might say food history has been consistently practiced as an academic subfield since the late fifteenth and sixteenth centuries, when a number of archaeologically minded discourses on the dining habits of the ancient world were written, the most celebrated by Stuckius, Boulenger, and Chacon. In the late eighteenth and early nineteenth centuries, nation states began to turn their attention to their own culinary traditions of the Middle Ages and Renaissance, eventually publishing editions of early cookbooks for historical study. Richard Warner's *Antiquitates Culinariae: Tracts on Culinary*

Affaris of the Old English of 1791 is an early example of such interest. In any case, food history is nothing new, even if it has only recently become a legitimate academic enterprise for professional historians. Moreover, today there are a significant number of historians, myself included, with academic appointments who identify their prime research field as food.

Distinct from these academic efforts is an entirely different endeavor, usually refered to as culinary history. Its practitioners are interested in using cookbooks to recreate culinary technologies as well as taste old recipes as a way to physically experience the past by proxy. There are also practical aesthetic reasons to cook old recipes. Tasting an approximation of a historic dish obviates the usual tendency to merely mock the flavor preferences of what most people construe as a strange and unfamiliar past. Through careful reconstruction of historic kitchens, obtaining appropriate ingredients and careful interpretation of recipes, the culinary arts of the past are revealed to be as sophisticated and complex as any other art form. The most adept of culinary historians have usually been found in 'living history' exhibits featuring live costumed cooks at historic sites such as Hampton Court in Britain or at Colonial Williamsburg and Plimoth Plantation in the U.S. Another impetus came from modern cookbook authors who sought to recover dying culinary traditions, which had been forgotten in the age of industrial food production. Historic recipes were part and parcel with a return to the land and an appreciation for flavors that speak of place, community, and timeless social values. Both the real ale campaign and efforts to reproduce farmhouse cheeses, along with numerous other products, were intitially historically motivated. Witness the proliferation of culinary history groups on both sides of the Atlantic, not to mention much of the Slow Food movement, whose inspiration is largely both nostalgic and gastronomic. Moreover, as historical recreation groups became more sophisticated, so too did their cooking expertise. Medieval and Civil War groups in the U.S. are sometimes among the most proficient and accurate of culinary historians.

Between the two approaches of food history and culinary history, however, few individuals have crossed over the boundary. This reflects a deep-seated prejudice in the academic tradition against 'getting your hands dirty' and delving into the actual physical practices of the past. Value and meaning is thought to be generated only by disembodied and presumably objective analysis. Subjects like food are studied only insofar as they reveal other topics, ultimately disconnected from and more important than food itself: subjects like class, race, gender, nationality. This attitude stretches all the way back to Plato, in fact (Curtin and Heldke). Thinkers comment upon and analyze practices, but they do not recreate the techne itself. Art historians should not mix paints and put brushes to canvas, literary scholars do not write sonnets, and historians of medicine unequivocably never play doctor.

At the same time, the so-called culinary *enthusiasts* or *amateurs* (both of which can be used in a pejorative sense, of course) rarely tackle socio-political theory or the cultural hermeneutics of food texts. They are interested in cooking. To a great extent their marginalization has been a matter of professional turf protection, as it is in so many fields. The distinction is much the same as between historians and antiquarians. It is assumed, wrongly, that because the historic cooks are not concerned with larger theoretical issues, their knowledge and skill are irrelevant for the scholarly discussion of food. Nothing could be farther from the truth.

Not only should this division between food historians and culinary historians be considered false and misleading, but it is actually dangerous for the food historian to proceed to say much at all meaningful about historic food practices without actually cooking. Cooking itself, procuring and processing food, moreover, has always been an integral part of the daily life of a significant proportion of the populace in any society, and therefore merits study, not only as a component of material culture but also as a way to understand people in the past and what was always a priority for every person every day – eating. Cooking is thus a kind of research methodology. Without it, critical analysis of cookbooks as historic texts is bound to go awry. Witness, for example, the many botched attempts to make sense of Apicius' text until very recently translated by a team of chef/ scholars (Grocock and Grainger, eds.).[1] What follows is a narrative account of several practical experiments undertaken in Renaissance cookery. What they have revealed will help illustrate why food studies in general could use a good dose of soot from the hearth.

First, a comparative illustration of how practice can inform theory may help to approach this topic obliquely. It is an example in many ways diametrically opposed to cooking, involving destruction and violence rather than nurture and creation, but thus all the more revealing. This example concerns a colleague of mine who specializes in military history. She has written about the personal experience of soldiers at war in the colonial era, not something one can easily imagine recreating with pleasure, though it is done by troupes of historical reenacters for entertainment and education. She was not very long ago invited at a conference to learn how to shoot an eighteenth-century musket. The image of a mild-mannered Scottish woman, ramming lead shot down a six-foot musket barrel is hard to imagine. But she did learn, and was drilled to reload and fire as quickly as possible. She later related to me that there was no possible way of understanding the terror of facing a line of muskets and reloading as fast as humanly possible, unless you had actually physically attempted to do it, stood choking in the blinding smoke and groped for your powder horn, while a Hessian charged at you with a bayonet. That is, the words of the soldiers themselves were only comprehensible in light of having physically experienced something similar. Why should the same not apply to the kitchen? The words of cookbook authors and food writers often only become meaningful when one follows their directions with ingredients, tools, and procedures that are as close as possible to the original. That is, to write intelligently about cooking practices and culinary texts, some cooking is logically requisite.

Approaching the historic cookery texts was undertaken, in a sense, the way an archaeologist might seek to understand a tool or process. That is, these

---

[1]   The translation by Grocock and Grainger should be compared with earlier unreliable attempts by Flower and Alföldi-Rosenbaum (1958) and Dommers (1936).

experiments did not involve merely trying to cook up a few old recipes using modern equipment and substituting ingredients when the originals became difficult to obtain. Adapting recipes in any way whatsoever tells us absolutely nothing about the past; it reveals only our modern preferences and prejudices. Or, to be blunt: the majority of historic cookbooks consisting of watered-down adaptations are completely useless for this kind of analysis. It would be like trying to learn about historic typography by studying fonts on a computer, or trying to understand Bach and how his audience perceived his music by hearing it performed on a piano, microphoned in a huge concert hall. That is, the technology, the techne, itself must be as authentic as possible to gain any really meaningful insights. Needless to say, the ingredients must be replicated exactly or the experiment is meaningless. This applies both to archaic spices as well as to animal breeds that have by and large changed in the modern era. For example, the lean industrial pig of recent decades cooks very differently from the fat porkers of the past, and historic recipes often fail for precisely this reason. In this case an heirloom breed reared using traditional methods is the only viable option. Where no direct equivalent could be found, the experiment could not be conducted.

Assay Number 1: Roasting

The first experiment concerns roasting, a word which today has an almost entirely different meaning than it did in the past. Trying to understand an historic recipe, or the physical experience of a cook, by what should properly be called baking in an oven is completely futile. First, baking is inherently easy. The food is placed in the oven, basted every now and then, removed, and served. Grilling is equally an entirely different procedure, and even a rotisserie mounted over a grill is not technically roasting. Roasting only really becomes clear when one listens very carefully to what cookbook authors were saying and follows their instructions to the letter, trusting not one's modern cooking sensibilities but those of the author. (It should be noted here that the art of proper roasting is not entirely moribund in Britain, as it is in the U.S.)

It should also noted that the goal here was foremost to analyze the experience of the professional cook as an academic topic, and only secondarily was there any interest in the taste of the food, at least initially. The experiment sprang from reading comments about the role of the professional cook in Bartolomeo Scappi's *Opera* of 1570 and specifically what a recipe on how to roast beef rib might reveal. This is the recipe:

> Per arrostire nello spedo la schiena di bove o di vaccina. (Book II Ch VI).

> Anchorche non sia in uso ponere nello spedo tal carne, pur io ritrovo, che si possano arrostire, & maggiormente quando saranno di meza età. Piglierasi dunque la schiena, & si compartirà in pezzi, che passino libre quatro, & ciascheduno di loro si farà stare per quattro hore in soppressa con sal trito, finocchìo over pitartamo, pepe ammaccato, & un poco d'aglio battuto, ponendoli

poi nello spedo senza essere rifatti, ne impillottati di lardo, & se vi si vorranno ponere alcuni rami di rosmarino per dentro, sarà in arbitrio, & similmente alcune cippole spaccate sotto nella ghiottela, lequali si cuoceranno con il grasso che da lor cascerà sopra, & cotte che saranno, si serviranno cosi calde con le cippole sopra, misticate con un sapore fatto d'aceto, mosto cotto, e spetierie communi.

To Roast on the spit the chine of steer or cow

Even though it is not in common usage to put this meat on a spit, still I have found, that you can roast it, and especially when it is of middling age. So take the chine and divide it into pieces, which are about four pounds, and each of them let stay for four hours pressed with ground salt, fennel or coriander, crushed pepper and a bit of pounded garlic, placing it on the spit without being parboiled, nor stuck with lard, but you can put some sprigs of rosemary between them, it will be as you like, and similarly some chopped onions beneath in the drip pan, which will cook with the drippings that fall over them, and when it's cooked, serve it hot with the onions on top, mixed with a sauce made of vinegar, cooked must and common spices.

The cut of meat in question, *schiena*, means back or chine (spine) to which is attached the ribs – a cut which ostensibly would today differ little from the past except perhaps in size and fat content, though Scappi does specify that this works with older animals. The placement of beef rib roast right at the start of the recipe section of the book suggests that this was a prestigious dish that a cook would have to execute fairly often, in this case for the papal court. That the procedure is also illustrated in the book further suggests the importance of spit roasting as typical of the Renaissance kitchen. Its prestige stems partly from the fact that it takes a great deal of fuel and manpower – someone must be hired to turn it. Though, the book does also show mechanical turnspits.

In the recipe, Scappi explains that it is not usual to spit roast this cut, but he finds that it can be roasted with excellent results, especially when the animal is mature. Thus this may well be a procedure he invented, or at least popularized. The meat is cut into 4-pound slabs; presumably he is segmenting an entire side. Then each cut is pressed, put under weights to marinate with a mixture of salt, fennel, or coriander, crushed pepper, and pounded garlic. The meat is then mounted on the spit 'senza essere rifatti' – without being redone (literally), though *rifare* here means to be parboiled, a very common procedure in medieval and early modern cookery. The very idea of parboiling beef before roasting it is completely foreign to modern cookery. To our sensibilities it would destroy the flavor – and most historical redactions skip it – which renders the final dish utterly different from the original. In fact parboiling does firm the meat so it stays on the spit, and it keeps the flesh moister because it seizes up and the juices do not leak out as it is being cooked. This procedure works with fowl too, and is a common practice in Asian cookery. This is a very good example of the need to follow the recipe exactly, especially when it makes little sense in modern culinary terms.

However, in any case, this recipe states that the ribs need not be parboiled – or larded, another practice to keep the meat moist. Larding is essentially little batons of fat knotted into the surface of the meat which melt and baste the meat as it roasts. So this recipe involves raw meat merely seasoned with a dry rub, and interspersed as Scappi says with sprigs of rosemary among the pieces of meat, if you like, and sliced onions in the dripping pan. Lastly, he says it is served with the onions and a sauce of vinegar, *mosto cotto* (cooked grape syrup), and typical spices (which in the sixteenth century would have been cinnamon, cloves, ginger, and perhaps sugar). This is essentially a good barbecue sauce.

So, then, how to really make sense of this recipe? One thing that is immediately apparent is that the roasting takes place beside a fire rather than over it, because there is a dripping pan to catch the fat and juices. This is a procedure adapted to cooking in front of a hearth. My own fireplace being not quite big enough, it seemed a fire outside would work better, and in fact there are illustations of this in Scappi as well. This would also facilitate cooking several dishes at the same time over or beside a large fire.

First a proper turn spit was required. This was forged with the help of friends in the art department and an acetylene torch. In the end, the 5-foot steel contraption closely resembled those illustrated in Scappi: a long rod with one sharp end and two bends in the other end and a wooden handle that rotates as the spit is rotated. About a foot down there were two fork prongs similar to a trident, to hold the meat in place. We also made two notched metal stanchions roughly 3 feet in height, which were driven into the ground, to hold the spit at either end and at variable heights, if desired, as it turned.

Next a pit was dug about 4 feet in depth and 4 feet in diameter and a fire built inside of oak wood. The beef roast was then mounted on the spit and set directly beside the roaring fire. Taking a cue directly from Scappi's illustrations, which show logs aflame and metal pots suspended over the fire and a roast beside it, the meat was not cooked over hot coals as on a modern barbecue. What became apparent immediately, apart from the fact that turning a spit is extremely laborious and sweaty, is that as the meat turns, the juices sear and then evaporate for just a few seconds without having a chance to burn. Thus the exterior becomes extraordinarily crispy and unctuous. There was maybe ¼ cup of drippings in the pan, just enough to brown the onions – but the vast majority of juices and flavor stayed inside the meat or had become part of the crust. The flavor was extraordinary, with only the subtlest hint of smoke, because there really was no smoke – certainly not as would be generated from a grill. To even greater surprise, the garlic never burned, it rather melded with the fennel and coriander in the crust. Also surprising is that in the time required to make this exterior crust, the meat was fairly well done inside, not in the least pink, but still full flavored, not in the least dried out, and extremely tender. It may be that the preference for rare meat in modern times is the result of baking meat, in which the juices merely seep out into the pan, and meat dries out if left to thoroughly brown. It also occurred to me, as a sudden revelation, that this may be precisely why meat-based sauces have come to dominate in classical French cookery after the eighteenth century. It is a way to put all the flavor back onto the meat in a sauce, rather than keeping it inside in the first place.

That is, insight into the development of flavor preferences over time only occurred after actually cooking a recipe, and in this case it may have been a change in technology that prompted the shift in culinary preference. The French devised a different way to cook beef because they were using indoor ovens and smaller cuts sauteed in pans rather than big cuts roasted in an open hearth, while the English, who still did traditionally proper roast beef, preferred it well done – not because they had poor taste but exactly the opposite: they were still using a tried and true technique. (Incidentally, the Italians, when they do roast, which is fairly uncommon, also do it beside a fire, and cook meat until well done.) What began as an exercise in culinary history actually revealed something about food history, the effects of technological change, the underlying reason for culinary differences, and deep-seated xenophobic antipathy between the French and English. It also revealed that cooking meat well was not the result of health concerns or any inherent fear of bloody meat. It had sound gastronomic origins.

Incidentally, subsequent roasting experiments, aided by a mechanical turnspit wound with a clock mechanism, have made possible many successful historic meals cooked before the fireplace indoors involving various cut of lamb, pork, and fowl. The same conclusion was confirmed: roasting can only truly be done with a spit before a fire, and it differs completely from other procedures which have informally borrowed the term 'roast'.

Assay Number 2: The Pipkin

This experiment concerns a fairly small clay cooking vessel called a pipkin. This is a round-bottomed bulbous pot with a narrow shoulder, slightly flaring rim, three small legs, and a hollow handle. Examples of these can be easily found in museums. Museums never explain the logic of the shape or why certain recipes call for the pipkin specifically. How one cooked in a pipkin was a mystery. In a modern kitchen we have become comfortable cooking in practically indestructable metal pots placed directly over high heat. The pikin, however, involved long slow cooking in a ceramic pot nestled in hot coals. The first problem was getting a pipkin. With many years experience making functional pottery and a ceramics studio under the kitchen, this obstacle did not seem insurmountable. However, my experience was limited to mid-range stoneware which can not be placed over direct heat lest the thermal shock (the result of one part of the pot heating more quickly than another) should cause it to crack, if not shatter violently. Ceramic cookware, historically, has always been made of low-fired earthenware. Experience cooking with a Spanish olla and other earthenware vessels for a while, with very positive results, was encouraging – but these are all flat-bottomed and designed to sit on a hub with a flame below (picture Velasquez's woman frying an egg). The pipkin is rounded, has legs, and, most importantly, was unglazed on the outside. My first thought was that this simply could not work – although traditional American Indian pots were also (completely) unglazed.

It was only after throwing a few pipkins that the logic of the shape became clear. The legs are simple enough; they hold the pot evenly over the coals so it will not tip over. The hollow handle open on the end also became obvious. You can just stick a rod in the end and lift the whole pot out of the fire. What I had not realized is that there is a structural reason for the rounded bottom too. It is not easy to throw such a shape, because the wheelhead is flat; the excess has to be trimmed off the bottom afterwards. But what became clear in cooking with these pots is that the flat-bottomed pipkins tended to crack, or pieces broke off of them. This has to do with the fact that there were differences in thickness between the walls and floor of the pot and structural weak points in the angled edges. With a rounded bottom, the pot heated evenly, the walls were uniformly thick, and it did not crack. The culinary history exercise revealed something about what one might have assumed were arbitrary or merely aesthetic choices. The demands of cooking dictated the form in this case. It also explains, incidentally, why medieval water jugs have a pinched foot around a rounded base: a flat bottom would explode in the kiln, for the same reason the flat pipkins cracked in the fire.

But there was also something more important, specifically about the unglazed surface. The clay itself is porous, soaks up liquids, and is a poor conductor of heat (unlike stoneware or porcelain). What that means is that when you place the pot over the coals, the pot walls stay relatively cool and keep the contents from boiling over or burning. You can basically fill it up, put it over hot coals, and forget about it. It simmers gently. And this explains why pipkins are often so small and recipes say you can cook a whole chicken in one (which you can). It also explains why nowhere in the culinary literature does anyone mention a pipkin boiling over, burning, or anything like that. It is the metal pots that they mention, for example fifteenth-century recipes explain how to remove the burnt flavor from a stew – because it has been cooked in a metal pot.

Here are the results of a complete experiment from beginning to end. The recipe is taken from *The Good Hous-wives Treasurie. Beeing a verye necessarie Booke instructing to the the dressing of Meates,* printed in London in 1588. It is a fascinating cookbook to start with, because it is written explicitly for women, running their own household. It is also a small and relatively cheap book, so we know it was probably made for the middling ranks of society rather than for grand courts with many servants. The quantities called for would also feed a family, so it is certain that this is not intended for a professional kitchen. Other clues also point to the social standing of the potential reader: sugar is called for in many of the recipes, as well as cinnamon and nutmeg, dried (and imported) currants (i.e., little raisins), dates, and orange peels, as well as exotic ingredients like rosewater and verjuice. That is, the potential reader is conversant with the latest culinary trends and has the money to afford these ingredients. Spices, dried fruits and nuts, and sugar were still fairly expensive, but they were being imported. So if you lived in London or a larger city, you could probably find these. Other clues suggest that the potential reader is fairly wealthy: ovens are called for in baking pies, and the aforementioned pipkin is often directed to be placed at the back of the hearth, under the chimney. So again, this all suggests an urban readership, primarily because there are no instructions at all for dealing with live animals, which are always found in cookbooks intended for manors and farms. The reader is clearly buying butchered meat.

These are some of the details a food historian may be able to sleuth out. But the recipes themselves are still very difficult to understand, and sometimes seem to defy all logic if you just read them. This is the case with a rabbit recipe, cooked in a pipkin. The verb 'to smear' has no recorded culinary use, and must refer to the unctuous texture of the final dish.

> How to smeare a Rabbet or a necke of Mutton (fol. A5)
>
> Take a pipkin, a porenger of water, two or three spoonefuls of Vergis, ten Onions pilled, and if they be great quarter them, mingle as much the Pepper and salte as will season them, and rub it upon the meat, if it be a rabbit put a piece of butter in the bellye and a peece in the brith, and a few currans if you will, stop your pot close and seeth it with a softe fier but no fier under the bottom, then when it is sodden serve it in upon soppes & lay a few Barberies upon the dish.

What is inscrutable from an initial reading is how a whole rabbit and 10 onions could fit in a little pot, why it isn't placed directly over flaming embers, why it doesn't burn with only about a cup of water, how it is stopped close, and – most importantly – what this could possibly taste like, and why the procedure is called 'to smear'? Following the recipe to the letter without trusting any modern culinary instincts revealed that the author knew exactly what she or he was doing. The whole rabbit was cut up, along with 10 small onions, and they did in fact all fit in the pipkin. The fairly simple spices, butter, and raisins were added, a mere porringer of water (about 3/4 cup), and the three spoons of verjuice, the juice of unripe grapes (using facsimiles modelled after fifteenth-century spoons dug from the Thames). A top was made of simple thick flour and water dough – the only practical way to seal the pot. It was then placed over hot coals and left to cook for about four hours. It did not burn at all, which was a surprise. The results were a revelation. Rather than the dry, boring, vaguely chicken-like texture of most modern rabbit recipes, this was unctuous, sweet, and well caramelized with a subtle sourness. It also, surprisingly, produced a great deal of what one must call gravy, which went perfectly over sops – i.e., slices of bread in a bowl. In other words, the recipe, which made absolutely no sense to the food historian, and might have been discarded as impractical or a 'bad' recipe, actually turned out to be magnificent, and it highlighted the unique cooking capabilities of the pipkin in a way that would never under any circumstances have worked in a metal pot over a modern range. This recipe only made sense when actually cooked as the author intended. Only with such an experiment could a scholar accurately annotate this recipe.

Assay Number 3: Danish Marzipan

This story derives from a talk given before the Greater Midwestern Food Alliance, the topic of which was the transmission of ideas and recipes using almonds from medieval Scandinavia to the nineteeth-century Midwest U.S. Chronologically in the middle of this span, the first printed Scandinavian cookbook was published in 1616, the *Koge-Bog: Indeholdendis et hundrede fornødene stycker*.[2] In it is a marzipan recipe that differs so much from our modern conception of marzipan that it seemed necessary to cook using the original tools and methods. The translation was produced with the invaluable aid of Henry Notaker.

LXXII. Martsipan at bage.

Stød skalede Mandel i en Morter/giff der vnder huit sucker oc Rosenvand/oc stød dette vel met huer andere/at det ey bliffuer fortyndt/men smuck tyck. Stryg dette paa Affladsblade/en Finger tyck/smuck jeffnet/som et Træ tellercken/leg det i en kaaberpande/som er smuck tør/giør det vnder en sact Ild/oc offuen paa et Kaaberlog/oc offuen paa samme Log ocsaa en sact Ild/lad det saa bagis. Naar det er bagit/saa ret an/oc bestrø det met Coriander/Anijss/etc.

Marzipan

Pound peeled almonds in a mortar/ add white sugar and rosewater/ and pound well together/ so it won't be too thin/ but suitably thick. Spread it on Affladsblade (Blotting paper?)/ one finger thick/ nicely leveled as a wooden plate/ put it in a copper pan that is well dry/ put it on a slow fire and put a copper lid on top and a fire on top of the lid also/ and let it be cooked. When it is cooked/ serve it and sprinkle with coriander, anis/ etc.

First, executing this involved blanching the almonds in boiling water to remove the outer peel. Next came pounding in a large mortar (from Punjab) which held 2 pounds of almonds comfortably. The process took about an hour or more until a smooth consistency was achieved with the sugar and rosewater added incrementally. One can appreciate the value of kitchen servants. The paste was spread on parchment paper, and the translation of the word *Affladsblade* was purely guesswork. No such word appears in Old Danish dictionaries, but other contemporary cookbooks do specify paper, and as we will see, it worked. The paper-lined paste went into a lidded pan onto slow burning coals for about 20 minutes, then was sprinkled with spices. The result was lightly browned, crunchy on the outside and soft on the inside, nothing like the modern product, but indeed more resembling a bread (March-pane as it was called in English) or a large cookie. Once again, without actually trying the recipe, it would have made no sense, and the *Affadsblade* would have remained a complete mystery. Moreover, one might have assumed there was some similarity between modern marzipan and the seventeenth-century century item, when in fact there is none.

---

[2]   For a Danish version on line, see Henry Notaker's Website: http://www.notaker. com/onlitxts/kogebog.htm

Assay Number 5: *Olla Podrida*

Experiment Number 5 was an attempt to make sense of a recipe that circulated throughout Europe from the late sixteenth century all the way to the eighteenth: the Olla Podrida. Not only is the name of the dish, meaning putrid pot (cognate with the French *pot pourris*) enough to put one off, but the odd concoction of discongruent ingredients alone is enough to inspire nausea and dread. The name presumably derives from the fact that the pot is cooked so long that everything falls apart and becomes indistinguishable. So the question was really to find out what all the fanatical interest was about. How is it that this dish rose to be one of the most popular in Baroque cookery, with examples garnished with lavish ingredients such as cockscombs, testicles, chestnuts, gooseberries, spiced, and perfumed with musk?

The other interesting feature of the recipe was its association with popular celebrations of Carnival or Mardi Gras, a day when all leftover meat had to be consumed prior to the fast of Lent. This may have explained the catch-all nature of the recipes, but its flavor and popularity still were elusive. How could a rustic hodge-podge become an elegant courtly dish?

The association of olla podrida with Carnival is made apparent in a series of silly short Carnival plays by Pedro Calderón (whose name means stew pot!), written in the early seventeenth century. They were performed privately, not publicly in the streets like earlier carnivals. One of these is *Carnestolendas (The Carnivalers)*, and another *Los Guisados (Stews)*, in which there is a succession of personified meat dishes – Menudo, Estofado, Don Mondongo – a blood sausage, Mrs. Abondiguilla (Meatball), and a Doña Olla Podrida who defends her endowments and inheritance, which include lamb and beef, bacon, and turnips. She says 'Mi dote (dowry) es grande: el tocino, el repollo (cabbage), los garbanzos, la berejena, el cardillo, las cebollas y los ajos'. All the stews get stabbed to death in the end (Calderón 1983, 409, lines 105–9).[3] In any case, it is a typical meat-based Carnival dish.

What did the Olla Podrida look like in Spain originally? First, as mentioned, it was usually considered a peasant dish to start with. That is the association made in Cervantes' *Don Quixote*. There is a fascinating scene in which Sancho Panza becomes governor of his own island (Ch XLVII) and he is about to eat dinner when a physician is standing next to him disapproving of all the dishes laid out on the table. Sancho points to a stew he sees:

> 'That big dish that is smoking farther off', said Sancho, 'seems to me to be an olla podrida, and out of the diversity of things in such ollas, I can't fail to light upon something tasty and good for me'.

> 'Absit', said the doctor; 'far from us be any such base thought! There is nothing in the world less nourishing than an olla podrida; to canons, or rectors of colleges, or peasants' weddings with your ollas podridas, but let us have none of them on the tables of governors, where everything that is present should be delicate and refined …'

---

[3]   The play is also available via www.cervantesvirtual.com

Notice that the doctor says an olla is good for peasants and rectors of colleges. And he then proceeds to recommend wafers and conserved quince, which of course is of no interest to Sancho.

What is fascinating in this case is that a recipe for olla podrida, exactly contemporaneous with Quixote, does appear in a cookbook by a college refectory cook. This is the *Libro del Arte de Cozina* written by Domingo Hernández de Maceras in 1607. He was the cook for the Collegio Mayor in Salamanca (which is also where Calderón went to study law in the 1620s), and although his students did not exactly suffer, I think it fairly accurately reflects ordinary eating habits, certainly more so than the courtly cookbooks of the same era like the *Arte de Cocina* by Martínez Montiño (1611).

> Cap LIII. Come se ha de hazer una olla podrida. (p.55)
>
> Para hazer una olla podrida, se le ha de echar carnero, vaca, tocino, pies de puerco, testuz, longanizas, lenguas, palomas, lavancos, liebre, lenguas de vaca, garvanços, ajos y nabos si es su tiempo, y la carne que cada uno quisiere; ha se de mezclar todo en una olla; y ha de cozer mucho: llevara sus especias y despues de bien cozida, se haran platos d ella, con mostaza de mosto, o dessotra, y por encima los platos echale perexil, proque perece bien, y es muy bueno.
>
> To make an olla podrida, you take lamb, beef, bacon, pig's feet, testuz (nape), lucanega sausages, tongues, pigeons, duck, hare, beef tongue, garbanzo beans, garlic and turnips in season, and whatever meat you want, and mix it all in an olla, and let it cook long in the olla. Add your spices, and when it is well cooked, make plates of it, with some mustard of grape must or other kind, and for each plate sprinkle parsley so it looks good, and is very good.

Cooking the recipe required a large fire pit similar to that mentioned in experiment 1 above, but of gentle coals into which a clay olla could be positioned. Since the recipe is fairly shorthand, some knowledge of ingredient preparation was required. The exact ingredients, following the author's suggestion, also appear variable, so not every item was considered absolutely necessary for the success of the finished dish. Most were included though. The ingredients began with lamb, in this case stew meat (shoulder), and beef stew meat (chuck), about 1/2 pound of each. Regular U.S. (streaky) bacon was used, though tocino could refer to a number of different cured pork products in seventeenth-century Spain. A pair of pig's feet entered in, but not the nape, which is merely a literal translation of a part that no butcher could identify, though some suggested collar. Portuguese *longaniça* plus an array of what in the US are politely referred to as squab were added, plus a rabbit cut up. The real challenge was the tongue, a whole beef tongue which was parboiled, skinned, cut up, and added to the pot. The garbanzo beans (chickpeas), turnips, and garlic are what really give a distinctive character to the dish.

With the exception of the pork products, the dish bears a certain relation to the Sephardic Jewish *adafina*, which was cooked the night prior to sundown before the Sabbath since Jews were forbidden to light fires from Friday sundown to Saturday sundown. The logic of the dish was that it could slowly cook all night on its own.

By the seventeenth century, observant Jews had been long expelled from Spain, though one is temped to see this as a survival, ironically enough, popular for the Catholic festival Mardi Gras.

After being cooked for about 5 hours, the meat in the pot was completely and utterly obliterated, and there was literally a gasp of disbelief when the top was removed before hungry diners (an elderly crowd at a theater benefit). It was, however, eaten avidly, and the flavors melded beautifully, with a deeply rich, smoky flavor accented with the chickpeas, which had browned nicely. The dish was, in a word, remarkably delicious, and not in flavor very different from a modern *cocido Madrileño*, though in that case it is cooked much quicker and the broth is served separate from the meat. It may nonetheless be a modern descendant changed with modern cooking implements and time restraints. One can certainly understand why this would have become a fashionable and elegant dish throughout Europe, but only after actually tasting it. The wild juxtaposed combination of meats and garnishes is esthetically perfectly Baroque in its complexity.

Assay Number 6: Garlic Soup

The following recipe was a simple experiment in aesthetics, a broadening of the palate comparable to tasting an exotic and unfamiliar dish for the first time. The mid sixteenth century, in gastronomic terms, was precisely such an exotic place, and one must expend considerable effort to understand the ubiquitous mingling of sugar with savory indredients. Sugar on pasta in Messisbugo's cookbook, sugar and cinnamon sprinkled on a chicken. These are actually approachable. But what of sugar in a savory soup, laden with garlic? Here is the recipe taken from the anonymous *Livre fort excellent de cuisine*, published in Lyon in 1555.

Souppe aux aulx

Pour une souppe aux aulx, prenes du vin blanc et mettes de la moelle de beuf dedans qui ayt este fort boully et des beaulx aulx aver prenes des aulx et les pilles & les mettes bouillir avec, prenes une perdrix ou deulx rosties et les mettes por quartiers parmy pour les espices gingemre & cloud de giroffle grant foyson de sucre Romarin hache bien dessye et laisser bien bouillir ensemble. Et a dresser des belles rostyes & les mettes au fond du plat mettes a servir de canelle bien peu ou du Gingembre.

For a soup of garlic, take white wine and place in some beef marrow which has been well boiled and some beautiful garlic. Take the garlic and peel it and place it to boil with it. Take a partridge or two roasted and quartered. For the spices, ginger, cloves, a great deal of sugar, finely chopped rosemary and let everything boil together well. Then arrange the lovely roast, place them in the bottom of the plate and serve with cinnamon or ginger.

Contrary to what one might expect, the great deal of sugar in the soup does not cloy, but accentuates the garlic, mellowing it, much as roasting garlic does, but rather than a deep caramelized flavor, one picks up the ginger and rosemary, which offset the roast fowl beautifully (as the author would say). It is not exactly the harmony one would expect from a classical French dish, in which a stock based on fowl would support the main ingredient. Rather, it is like counterpoint. Different flavors can all be heard together with none dominating. They vie with each other creating textural contrasts, exactly the same way sixteenth-century century music and mannerist art achieve the same effect. In other words, cooking this dish revealed nothing new, but actually tasting it offered invaluable insights into why sixteenth-century diners appreciated sugar in contexts from which we can only recoil today. The experiment revealed that the same aesthetic choices that inform music and painting were also at play in gastronomy.

Assay Number 7: *Escabeyg*

A final story, one that illustrates why cooking is a valuable research tool. This experiment concerns recipes themselves and the importance of following directions carefully. We tend to think that cookbook authors of the past were imprecise or vague because they had not yet learned to use scientific measurements or cooking times, or that they were written in a kind of shorthand for professionals who understood the basic procedures, so they had no need to be explained the way modern cookbook authors do. In fact, much of the reason historic recipes look so bizarre is because either people are not willing to follow them exactly so they end up with something completely different that does not taste good (for example a tansy, which is basically a cut up green omelet, one well-respected food historian changed to a pancake 'since small pancakes seem more attractive than a cut up green omelet'. This of course ignores the fact that it was cut up so you could eat it with your fingers (Like tamago egg sushi). Or modern readers are led astray when they look at a recipe and decide there is no way this could possibly work and then adapt it to suit their own tastes or equipment or culinary experience. A case in point is the ubiquitous 'snow' that shows up in the cookbooks of every Western European country in the sixteenth century. Some recipes say to mix egg whites and cream and beat it up with flavorings until it whips into a frothy mass. Even the most rudimentary of basic modern cookery informs us that there is no way that could work, and a modern reader easily assumes that the authors really meant beat the eggs and cream separately and fold together afterwards. In fact, that is not what they meant. And it does actually work. The lesson to be learned is that cookbook authors actually knew what they were talking about, and to learn from them one has to be willing to trust them implicitly. Usually when something does not work, it is because you have misread the instructions. (Or, more rarely, it is a typesetter's or translator's mistake, which does happen.)

This example is a bizarre medieval Catalan *escabeyg* from the fourteenth-century *Livre de Sent Sovi*. Solicitous care was taken with this recipe, partly because of the difficulty of the language, but also because it sounded absolutely revolting, and the dish, however it turned out, would be served to a group of history students at the inauguration of a new honor society chapter. There is always something appealing about a captive audience, but young and often picky undergraduates made this a double challenge.

Pex Ffrit ab Escabeyg (p. 207)

Ages de bon pex e ffrig-lo. E puyx ages ceba menut tellada, e soffrig-la ab olli. Puy prin primerament pa torrat mullat en vinagre, e de la polpa del pex ab salsa, e pique-u hom bé ab de la ceba soffrita. E puy, quant bé serà piquat, destrempa-ho a aygua calda, e va en la casola on és la seba soffrita; e met-hi un poch de vinagre per asaborir. Puy quant bull, va sobre l pex en telladors. e qui hi vol jurvert perbullit, pots-ho-hi piquar, e avellanes tenbé.

Take good fish and fry it. And then take onions chopped small and fry in oil. Then take bread first toasted and soaked in vinegar, and some flesh of the fish with spices, and pound it well with the fried onions. Then when it is well pounded, moisten with hot water, and put it into the pan where the onion cooked and add a little vinegar to flavor. Then when it boils, pour it over the fish in a platter. And if you want, some parboiled parsley and also hazelnuts.

My first instinct was to ignore the directions and try something vaguely similar that people would eat: perhaps breading and frying the fish, though it does not say to do that. Or maybe using buttered breadcrumbs and scattering them on the top, though this is supposed to be a Lenten dish, so there is no butter or animal products in it. The idea came to me to marinate the fish in the vinegar, like *escabeche*, which is the descendant of this dish. Instead, the recipe was followed to the letter: the fish was fried and arranged on a platter. Then the bread was toasted and soaked, some of the fish was added, vinegar, and the fried onions and spices (cinnamon, pepper, and ginger – which is typical of this period) and everything was dumped in the mortar and pounded for about a half an hour until it looked exactly like brown vomit. This was poured over the fish, sprinkled with hazelnuts and parsley (parboiled – or blanched so it actually keeps its color when set out). In the end, it did not look quite as revolting as the recipe sounded. It disappeared within a few minutes. The lesson learned is that if a recipe does not work, no one would remember it or put it on paper. That only happens nowadays – when there are professional cookbook writers (who do not always test recipes as they should) as opposed to cooks who recorded their extensive experience in the kitchen. That is, to learn about historic culinary procedures, we must trust what is on the page.

In conclusion, experiments that might have seemed pedestrian or a messy waste of time yielded valuable historical information about cooking technology, the development of taste preferences over time (and perhaps something about what the food actually tasted like – it is definitely not strange or inedible). There were also valuable insights to be gained into the labor involved for cooks, and of course how to interpret historical documents like cookbooks and other food texts. This was information not just how, but why things in the past were cooked as they were, and these experiments provided useful examples of why culinary history and food history should be more closely aligned, if not one and the same.

Works Cited

Anon. 1555. *Livre fort excellent de cuisine*. Lyon. Olivier Arnoulet.

————. 1588. *The Good Hous-wives Treasurie. Beeing a verye necessarie Booke instructing to the the dressing of Meates*. London. Edward Allde.

————. 1616. *Koge-Bog: Indeholdendis et hundrede fornødene stycker*. Kiøbenhaffn (Copenhagen). Salomone Sartorio.

————. 1979. *Livre de Sent Sovi*. Ed. Rudolf Grewe. Barcelona. Editorial Barcino.

Athenaeus. *The Deipnosophists*. 1927. Trans. Charles Burton Gulick. London. Heinemann.

Calderón de la Barca, Pedro. 1983. *Entremeses, jácaras y mojigangas*. Edición, introducción y notas de Evangelina Rodríguez y Antonio Tordera. Madrid. Castalia.

Cervantes, Miguel de. 1999. *Don Quijote*. Ed. Diana de Armas Wilson; Trans. Burton Raffel. New York. W.W. Norton.

Curtin, Deane W., and Lisa M. Heldke, eds. 1992. *Cooking, Eating and Thinking*. Bloomington. Indiana University Press.

Dommers, Joseph Vehling, trans. 1936; repr. London, 1977. *Apicius: Cookery and Dining in Imperial Rome*. Chicago. W. M. Hill.

Flower, Barbara, and Elizabeth Alföldi-Rosenbaum, trans. 1958. *The Roman Cookery Book. A Critical Translation of 'The Art of Cooking'*. London and Toronto. Harrap.

Grocock, Christopher, and Sally Grainger, trans. 2006. *Apicius: a critical edition with an introduction and an English translation of the Latin recipe text Apicius* Totnes. Prospect.

Maceras, Domingo Hernández de. 1999. *Libro del Arte de Cozina, 1607*. Salamanca. Ediciones Universidad de Salamanaca.

Martínez Montiño, Francisco. 1763. *Arte de Cocina, 1611*. Barcelona: Maria Angela Marti.

Scappi, Bartolomeo. 2002. *Opera, 1570*. Bologna. Arnaldo forni.

Warner, Richard. 1791. *Antiquitates Culinariae: Tracts on Culinary Affaris of the Old English*. London. R. Blamire.

Chapter 5
Distillation:
Transformations in and out of the Kitchen

Wendy Wall

> Distilling is beautiful. First of all because it is a slow, philosophic, and silent
> occupation, which keeps you busy but gives you time to think of other things,
> somewhat like riding a bike. Then, because it involves a metamorphosis from
> liquid to vapor (invisible), and from this once again to liquid; but in the double
> journey, up and down, purity is obtained, an ambiguous and fascinating condition
> (Primo Levi, 57–8).

I start with what might seem to be a detour around the topic of the kitchen, for
I begin with the beginning of Shakespeare's *Sonnets*, a well-known literary text
that famously ushers the reader into unexpected terrain. Instead of asserting ardent
desire, as was common in sonnet sequences of the day, the speaker in the opening
lines of the first sonnet declares: 'From fairest creatures we desire increase / That
thereby beauty's rose might never die'.[1] The dilemma that these sonnets describe is
mortality, with tyrannical time threatening being and beauty. Against the possibility
of 'bareness everywhere', the speaker seeks measures for insuring plenitude and
duration, one of which is expressed – in sonnets 5 and 6 – through reference to the
trope of distillation. After personifying summer as a being lured into the withering
cold of winter, in Sonnet 5 he states:

> Then were not summer's distillation left
> A liquid prisoner pent in walls of glass,
> Beauty's effect with beauty were bereft,
> Nor it nor no remembrance what it was.
> But flowers distill'd, though they with winter meet,
> Leese but their show, their substance still lives sweet.

Holding at bay death and decay, distilling provides a form of remembrance in
which the flower's mere trappings – its 'effect' or 'show' – can be discarded so that
its substance might persevere. Using characteristically complex double negatives,
this sonnet returns to the 'rose' whose beauty the first sonnet sought to increase.
The next sonnet continues the trope as the speaker somewhat desperately urges
the beloved to undertake the sexually suggestive action of being distilled: the
friend should 'make sweet some vial' and 'treasure ... some place', phrases that

---

[1]   All quotations of Shakespeare's *Sonnets* and plays are from Shakespeare 1974.

vaguely call forth images of bodily receptacles. Distillation seems a metaphor for reproduction, with the 'liquid prisoner' from Sonnet 5 now back-projected as potent semen that can reduplicate fathers into the signifying children that will bear the parents' memory. The beloved should act as the agent and object of distillation, refiguring his own 'substance' so as to 'still' live, like the rose: sweet, remembered, beautiful, fair. As such, these sonnets hint at the magical beauty of distillation that Primo Levi describes in my epigraph.

In these initial sonnets, reproduction is complemented and then rivaled by the immortality offered specifically by poetry: 'All in war with Time for love of you', the speaker boldly declares in Sonnet 15, 'As he takes from you, I ingraft you new'. If we draw from one of the sonnets' own rhetorics, we might say that they self-reflexively declare their graphic and distillatory power. In a later sonnet, number 54, the speaker assures the beloved that 'verse distills your truth': the limbeck of poetic practice can secure an essence in part by freeing it from the limitations of single form. The printed poems that the reader holds thus enact and document the immortalization praised by the speaker. They have been, it seems, distilled, with beauty playing a role slightly different than the one Levi imagined as produced by the very process of distillation. It was, of course, conventional for writers to declare poetry as a tool in the war against time. But how might poetic immortalization have been imagined *as* distillation in early modern terms?

By this point you might wonder what sonnets have to do with the kitchen. In this essay, I seek to restore a neglected context for understanding distillation – that of early modern domestic labor. This issue is signaled in Ralph Knevet's 1631 play *Rhodon and Iris*, in which a serving woman complains about the lengths that her mistress goes to in order to catch a man. Eglantine comments: 'With limbecks, viols, pots, her Closet's fill'd / Full of strange liquors by rare art distilled' (E3v). In the intimate closet of the upper middling home, a space that has itself been the nodal point for critical claims about privacy, property, and interiority, there exists something 'strange' that women concoct through a rare and yet domestic art; it seems common, that is, for women to have limbecks at home. What might it matter – meaning to render material or show significance – to locate distillation within the kitchen? Might it refine our understanding of inscribed immortalization? Or allow us to see that debates prominent in and around canonical literary texts – about artifice and nature, or substance and form – had a correlate in the practice and conceptualization of household tasks in the period?

Art and Nature: Kitchen Style

The science of distillation involves heating and cooling a substance so as to vaporize and concentrate the properties of a given entity. It is a method of separating chemical substances based on the fact that entities vaporize at different temperatures. The most popularly recognized apparatus for distillation in modern times is the 'still', which largely is used to make alcoholic beverages. But evidence from Greece, Mesopotamia, and Pakistan indicate that distillation has been used for many purposes (e.g., industrial, pharmaceutical, and chemical). Since Persian experimenters created the limbeck (or alembic) around 800 AD well into the early modern period, it remained the most common apparatus for distillation.

Most critics read Shakespearean sonnets' references to distillation as taking meaning primarily from the discourse of alchemy, a somewhat esoteric male learned art with a particular history. Although people had distilled alcohol in ancient times, it only appeared in alchemical literature around 1300. Writers focusing on distillation alchemy included thirteenth-century friars Roger Bacon (*The Mirror of Alchemy*) and Raymond Lull (*The Book Concerning the Secrets of Nature*); fourteenth-century friar John of Rupescissa (*Concerning the Fifth Essence* and *The Book of Light*); fourteenth-century physician Petrus Bonus of Ferrara (*The Precious Pearl*); and sixteenth-century teacher Andreas Libavius (*Alchemy*).[2] While their texts vary in emphasis, each outlines the technical chemical procedures that enable substances to be transmuted into a purified and mystical form that might prolong life (what Bacon called 'magisteries') (Moran 10). Deeply invested in an Aristotelian natural philosophy, medieval alchemy was largely metallurgical; that is, it typically traded in magical elixirs that promised to break down and reconstitute the properties of metals, often with a particular focus on mercury and sulphur. One of Shakespeare's later sonnets, number 119, negatively values the mystical properties of alchemical distillation, merging it with a well-known mythological figure. When the speaker claims to have drunk siren tears 'Distilled from limbecks foul as hell within', he suggests the supernatural dimension of alchemy. Whether working in a utilitarian craft tradition or in more mystical magical systems, alchemists largely chose not to distill substances as mundane as the roses mentioned in Shakespeare's early sonnets.

Unlike alchemists, medicinal distillers tended to downplay the search for the Philosopher's Stone or the Grand Elixir and concentrate instead on the possible curative properties of common herbs and plants. Practiced by physicians and apothecaries well into the seventeenth century, the male craft of medicinal distillation was a knowledge made available to a larger public through books such as Hieronymus Brunschwig's 1527 *The vertuose boke of distyllacyon of the waters of all maner of herbes,* which inaugurated a set of treatises in the sixteenth and seventeenth centuries. Brunschwig, who based his knowledge on the 'thirty years study ... of the most ... famous master of physic', offers technical instructions for readers accompanied by numerous illustrations documenting the often cumbersome laboratory equipment required for the job. Konrad Gesner's *The new Jewell of Health* (translated into English in 1576) similarly served as an encyclopedia of the different practices and different furnaces to be used in the 'secret' art of distillation. In the late sixteenth and early seventeenth centuries, distillation was represented as a requisite skill in pharmacology books and books of secrets, texts that taught the art of creating wondrous medicines, oils, tinctures, extracts, dyes, inks, and balsams.

---

[2]   My description of alchemical distillation is drawn from Moran 8–36.

Yet, while distilling remained an ongoing practice among apothecaries and professionals interested in herbal medicines, a wave of popular printed domestic manuals and recipe books in late sixteenth-century England newly classified distillation as female domestic work. The title page to the earliest published books of culinary, medical, and household recipes routinely advertised distillation as something that every good housewife should know.[3] Rather than delving into arcane or mystical chemical processes, recipe books offered practical advice on how to modify wines and waters so as to create medicines and foodstuffs. One of the most popular of such books was Hugh Plat's decorative 1602 *Delightes For Ladies, to Adorne their Persons, Tables, Closets, and Distillatories*, which was reprinted in numerous editions throughout the seventeenth century. Ornamented with designed borders and small enough to fit into a pocket, Plat addresses women who enjoy leisure and shopping as much as arduous housework. Catering to upwardly mobile urban women, Plat groups his 'delights' into four rubrics – on conserving, cookery, cosmetics, and 'Secrets in Distillation'. In the 25 recipes in the distilling section, the reader learns how to concoct various spiced wines (some flavored with vegetables) and numerous waters which could draw out the properties of herbs and flowers. Notably, Plat includes seven different recipes for distilling roses and two others that can be used to transform any flower; for Plat, roses are one of the most prominent substances in the household distillatory.

Domestic distillation shared with alchemy the translation of solids into liquid and vaporous forms through alternate heating and cooling, often using alcohol as the medium for achieving this action. The goal was the separation of the essence from waste matter, often figured as a corporeal residue. Plat's instructions for how to extract what he terms the substance's 'true spirit' or the 'blood' from its leftover waste matter is evidenced in his recipe for 'the spirit of spices', where the reader is to create an oil by bottling spices for a month and then seething them in a limbeck. Plat writes:

> Distill with a gentle heat either in balneo [vessel of boiling water] or ashes the strong and sweet water where with you have drawen oils of cloves, mace, nutmegs, juniper, Rosemarie, &c. after it hath stoode one moneth close stopt, and so you shall purchase a most delicate spirit of each of the saide aromaticall bodies. (E2v Recipe 3)

In Plat's vocabulary, spices constitute gross mass bodies that can be transformed into delicate spirits. A later recipe promises to make honey 'yeelde his spirit by distillation' (E8r Recipe 13). Steeped in the corporeal vocabulary that alchemy typically used, distillation could volatize substances so as to expel indelicate elements. Brunschwig explains that distillation involved 'a purifying of the grosse from the subtyll and the subtyll from the grosse, each separately from other to the

---

[3]   See, for instance, Dawson, title page. For examples of other distillation recipes in early modern books, see Anon., *A Closet for Ladies* 48–52; and Partridge, *Treasurie* 1–58. Best offers a helpful introduction to distilling in his edition of Markham (xl–xlii).

entent that the corruptyble shall be made incorruptyble and to make the materyall immateryall' (A1r).

Household manuals that targeted country estate dwellers rather than cosmopolitan ladies also identified distillation as a domestic practice and included descriptions of types of stills to be used (e.g., pewter, wood, or glass). Gervase Markham's comprehensive reference guide, *The English Huswife: Containing the Inward and outward Vertues which ought to be in a compleate Woman. As her skill in Physicke, Surgerie, Extraction of Oyles, Cookery, Banqueting-stuffe, Ordering of great Feasts, Preserving of all sorts of Wines, Conceited Secrets,* [and] *Distillation...,* seeks to identify household management as the core to a national ethic based on thrift. In a world in which the housewife is expected to tend the dairy, make cheese, and brew beer, she must also be concerned with vaporizing and condensing complex waters and wines, an art fundamental for her primary domestic responsibility – household healthcare. Markham designates physic as the chief principal 'vertue' that the housewife is to display (4), and he includes numerous distillation recipes for healing waters, including distillations of sage, radishes, endive, sorrel, roses, rosemary, strawberries, cloves, and aluminum. Markham urges the housewife to 'furnish herself of very good Stils, for the distillation of all kindes of Waters, which Stils would either bee of Tinne, or sweet Earth; and in them shee shall distill all sorts of waters meete for the health of her Houshold' (129). The title page to Hannah Woolley's later manual *The Queene-like Closet or Rich Cabinet* pictures women working with the type of distilling equipment that Markham recommends for the home.

In assigning women the task of distillation, Markham and Plat followed the lead of Thomas Tusser, who scripted the most famous almanac-based domestic guide for the small farmer and housewife in the early modern period. Tusser's handy *One Hundred Points of Good Husbandry* expanded in its many editions to *Five Hundreth Pointes of Good Husbandrie*. Organized principally by the season, *Five Hundreth Pointes* provides a helpful calendar of tasks rendered in short jingling rhymed couplets designed for easy memorization. Each month offers an abstract of the duties that the chapter addresses, followed by tetrameter elaborations. His list of tasks for March includes a list of 'Herbs to still in sommer', including blessed thistle (which strengthens memory, sharpens the wits, and prevents madness), betany (primarily for headache but also good for dog bites and deafness), dill (an expectorant and cure for hemorrhoids), eyebright (for eye problems and purging phlegm), fumitory (a laxative), and hyssop (an ingredient used to cure cough, gout, pleurisy, and jaundice), mint (for an overly hot liver or dry hands), and roses (an all purpose ingredient used in cures for headache, back pain, vomiting, eyesores, and mouth cankers (Tusser 76). In recommendations for work to be undertaken in May, Tusser offers a revealing ditty: 'Wife as you will / Now plie your still' (86). Vigorously working, or 'plying', her still, the housewife undertakes an indispensable part of housewifery. The casual phrase, 'as you will' (chosen most probably in order to rhyme with 'still'), hints at the freedom of choice that might be exercised through housewifery in tandem with its goal of honest industry. Tusser's sense that the reader will customize her practice is not unusual; household guides routinely pepper their instructions with assurances that the reader will have the liberty of tailoring tasks to suit her desires (Wall 42–58). Tusser's poem foregrounds the commonly perceived combination of energetic labor and exercise of choice vested in female housework. Choosing to design experiments as she 'will' and exerting her 'will', the early modern housewife exercised a certain degree of autonomy and authority in domestic work.

As we see from the many household advice books published in the period, even the housewife with few resources was expected to distill complex drinkable waters, culinary seasonings and flavorings, skin care products, medicinal cures, and household 'sweeteners' to void the body and air of pestilence (soaps, pomanders, and perfumes). Distillation figures most crucially in domestic healthcare, with rosewater serving as an essential staple for concoctions that 'cooled' fevers and voided bad vapors. Most readers of Shakespeare's *Sonnets* assume, however, that the distilled immaterial prisoner extracted from the rose must be perfume, something cosmetic and readily collapsible into the aesthetic. All major editions of Shakespeare's *Sonnets* available to students gloss the word 'distillation' as perfumes made from flowers. In part this assumption is based on the fact that a later sonnet, number 54, specifically describes the products of distilled roses as 'sweetest odors'. In the earlier two poems, however, distilled roses are not specified as sweet smelling dematerialized aesthetic objects readily analogous to poetry's literary effects. Instead, they would have been seen, as these recipe books reveal, as highly functional entities used in a variety of ways to prevent natural decomposition. Rosewater 'comfortheth and strengtheth and coleth the braynes the harte, the stomake and the pryncipall members & defendeth them from dyssolvynge', one text promises of its distilled rosewater (Brunschwig R1r). Plat makes sure that his reader knows that rosewater is the basis for numerous syrups and waters; he advises, 'Stampe the leaves, and first distill the juice being expressed and after distill the leaves … and so you shall dispatch more with one Stil then others do with three of foure stils. And this water is every way … medicinable …, serving in all sirrups, decoctions, &c. sufficiently' (E9r–E9v Recipe 15).

Tusser similarly emphasizes the pragmatic value of distillation:

> The knowledge of stilling is one pretty feat,
> The waters be wholesom, the charges not great.
> What timely thou gettest, while summer doth last
> Think winter will help thee to spend it as fast. (108)

Tusser locates distilling within the circuit of getting and spending that saturates kitchen work. 'Getting' (closely aligned semantically in early modern texts with 'begetting') is driven by a seasonal imperative: the storing of bounty from summer's harvest provides for winter's expenditures. Tusser's vocabulary resonates with the 'husbandry' metaphors that pervade the first poems in Shakespeare's *Sonnets*: the beloved is urged to be a good husband, that is, to manage his sexual and other resources; wise expenditure enables value, namely beauty. The sonnets deploy the word 'use' in outlining this dilemma: 'unused' beauty is an 'abuse' of resources, usury, in fact (see Greene). In his guide, Tusser similarly sees timely spending as allowing summer to last; stilling stores value by restoring the humoral balance of bodies but also by recreating natural products for better use. Distilled flowers, spices, and herbs, it seems, produced more than perfume.

Delights for Ladies

Distillation often took meaning from the practice of confectionary to which it was commonly conjoined in recipe books and in the kitchen space in which each was conducted. Both confectionary and distillation concerned the technical transformation of natural substances through artificial means, as Plat's preface to his recipe book *Delights for Ladies* suggests. Addressing 'all true Lovers of Arte and Knowledge', Plat offers a poetic manifesto outlining housewifery's exquisite power to overgo the limits of nature, an unusually literary feature for a recipe book. He writes his text, he states, not with the typical ink of 'coppres, or with gall', but with a distilled substance: 'Rosewater is the inke I write withall', he declares, before explaining that he turns from martial activity to dessert making, offering 'sweets' to the 'sweetest creatures', his female readers (Plat A2v):

> To sweetest creatures that the earth doth beare:
> These are the Saints to whom I sacrifice
> Preserves and conserves both of plum and peare.
> Empaling now adew, tush marchpaine wals,
> Are strong enough, and best befits our age:
> Let pearcing bullets turne to sugar bals,
> The Spanish feare is husht and all their rage.
> Of Marmelade and paste of Genua,
> Of musked sugar I intend to wright,
> Of Leach, of Sucket, and Quidinea,
> Affording to each Lady, her delight. (A2v)

Offering his services to ladies in a highly literary and rhetorical gesture, Plat suggests affinities between his sweet clientele, aesthetically delightful text, and sugary recipes. Satirizing the superficiality of a world as flimsy as marzipan, he nevertheless praises domesticity, in mock epic intonations, as worthy of sacrifice (see Hall). Plat promises that his recipes are designed to enhance the work that will ensure women's pleasure.

As part of this mission, Plat proclaims housewifery's power to rival nature:

> I teach both fruites and flowers to preserve,
> And candy them, so Nutmegs, cloves, and mace:
> To make both marchpane paste, and sugred plate,
> And cast the same in formes of sweetest grace.
> Each bird and foule, so moulded from the life,
> And after cast in sweete compounds of arte,
> As if the flesh and forme which nature gave,
> Did still remaine in every lim and part (A2v–A3r).

Can the housewife craft sugar foodstuffs that are so convincing that the natural 'flesh and forme' seems to 'remaine in every lim and part'? How can nature 'remain' in something synthetic? What does natural 'form' mean in this context? In Plat's language, artifice seems to restore life to inanimate desserts such that they partake of the essence of the thing they represent. Plat's word 'lim', meaning both a body part ('limb') and the act of adorning with a paintbrush ('to limn'), only further collapses the difference between a capon and its sugary representation in 'compounds of arte'.

Plat's witty confectionaries were examples of the sugared simulacra of reality that housewives of the middling sort were enjoined to make at the end of the sixteenth century, as they were invited to create scaled-down versions of the elaborate sugar sculptures spectacularly displayed at medieval and Renaissance banquets. Plat revels in describing the 'rare and strange device[s]' that comprise desserts, or 'banqueting' dishes, as they were called (B4r). Using sugar plate or marzipan, the housewife was to 'print' foodstuffs into the shape of animals, emblems, implements, cards, saucers, dishes, coats of arms, or edible letters. In one such recipe, 'A most delicate and stiffe sugar past whereof to cast Rabbets, Pigeons, or any other little birde or beast, either from the life or carved molds', the reader is taught how to use rosewater and isinglass (material from the bladder of a fish) to form a glutinous substance that can be molded to form rabbits or birds (B3v Recipe 10). The recipe even shows the housewife how to dredge the creature with a combination of breadcrusts, cinnamon, and sugar so it will seem to be roasted. In this way, Plat explains, 'a banquet may be presented in the forme of a supper' (B4r Recipe 10). Dessert, that is, mimics the savory meat course, wittily reconstituting, in faux form, what has already been eaten. Capitalizing on the representational capacity of food, confectionary could become a 'thinkpiece' on matter and natural form. Not only is nature replicated through artifice, but rituals of eating heralded by moralists as establishing social place through decorum, are mimed as part of the conceit.

In one manuscript recipe book handed down from a mother to her daughter, Mary Granville includes instructions for creating marzipan-shaped flowers (called 'violet cakes') coloured with violet juice, which are made out of beaten violets. Put 'as much powder of the violets thereof as will colour it according to your owne desire', she instructs, before offering other recipes for how to dye the material to look like different flowers (Granville 50). A similar recipe, 'To make Paste of Violets, or any kinde of Flowers' appears in a recipe book entitled *The Ladies Cabinet Opened and Enlarged*, where the reader is directed:

> Take your flowers, pick them and stamp / them in an Alabaster Morter; then steep them two hours in a Sawcer of Rose-water, after strain it, and steep a little Gumme Dragon [tragachant, adragant, a resin extracted from a Persian plant] in the same water; then beat it to paste, print it in your Moulds, and it will be of the very colour and taste of the Flowers; then gild them, and so you may have every Flower in his own colour and taste; better for the mouth then any painted colour. (30–31)

Here the flower is crushed in a mortar, condensed into a liquid, congealed with a gummy substance, and then remade into the form of a flower. If a violet is used to create and scent a paste that is then pressed into the shape of a violet, what is its relationship to being a violet? Is it a copy? What type of mimesis is at work? Although the writers of these recipe books did not explicitly comment on this quandary, the fact that the violet (or other flower) is reconstituted into another type of violet suggests that confectionary played on the inextricable line between inscription and inscribed matter, an early modern notion of 'writing' that Juliet Fleming has tutored us to understand in other arenas (see Spiller xv–xvii; Fleming 2001). In devising what one cookery book says are candied roses that look 'as naturally as if they grew upon the Tree', recipe books posed the domestic quandary of the artificial yet unpainted object, a natural piece of art (Anon 1608, 17).

For Plat, the mimetic force of confectionary is tied to the kitchen's power to provide a durable substitute for nature. In the prefatory poem, he writes passionately that he can stop the 'chrystall frost' from nipping the tender grape; in fact he asks the reader to visualize this triumph in the material book, which appears to show nature distilled: 'Yet heere *behold* the clusters fresh and faire' that are 'heere from yeere to yeere preserved, / And made by arte with strongest fruits to last' (Plat A3r emph. mine). Artichokes and quinces are 'here maintain'd and kept most naturally', positioned next to the waters and oils filling ladies 'stillatories' (Plat A3r). These items are paradoxically kept 'naturally' 'by arte'. Much as the speaker in Shakespeare's *Sonnets*, Plat is concerned with the way that humans might intervene in natural temporal cycles so as to thwart decay. Yet in Plat's narrative, it is explicitly the housewife who preserves essences, albeit for the practical purpose of consuming fruit out of season and from year to year. In his suggestion that confections substitute for reality and that art fulfills nature, Plat grapples with nothing less than the issues of mimesis that preoccupied thinkers such as Plato, Aristotle, and Sidney (a subject taken up as well by alchemists).[4]

While most recipe books do not explicitly meditate upon housewifery's power to deploy art to supplement nature, this issue creeps into cookery books in the many recipes that claim to preserve natural products beyond their expiration or to fortify human beings against mortality. Numerous books assure readers that strawberries, artichokes, quinces, or barberries can be made to 'keep' all year or that medicinal syrups will last many years and prolong life. As such, recipe books locate humans in the mortal world of fruits and animals even as they attempt to thwart the natural cycles that erode living things. Cookbook writer John Partridge announces in a prefatory poem that his recipes will 'maintaine life, & kepe ye yong, the cheefest thing ye crave' (A1v). Partridge's recipe for Gascoigne wine, distilled with ginger, cinnamon, and nutmeg, promises to calm spirits, contract sinews, and heal a variety of problems – including palsy, barrenness, worms, gout, toothache, stomachache, and bad breath. It allowed the notable Dr. Stephens, Partridge notes,

---

[4]   According to Newman, alchemy could involve a profound meditation on mimesis and the relationship between art and nature (111–14). See also Smith.

to live to the ripe old age of 96 (F8v). In its ongoing struggle against the negative effects of temporality, domestic work was distilling writ large.

Plat's pragmatic claims for distilling positively value the pejorative discourse around female cosmetics that saturates early modern writing. In literary texts, accusations of painted women as the ultimate emblem of duplicity crop up with great frequency. Hamlet, for instance, famously punctuates his meditation about the ultimate decay of the flesh in the graveyard with a call for a woman to understand the futility of her own 'paint' (5.1.192). In *Rhodon and Iris*, this common tirade against cosmetics is explicitly linked to distillation. Clematis complains that her mistress Eglantine relies on potions, lotions, salves and liquors to falsify her body:

> Sweet waters she distils, which she composes
> Of flowers of Oranges, Woodbine or Roses:
> The vertue of Jesmine and three-leav'd grasse,
> She doth *imprison* in a brittle glasse
> With Civet, Muske, and odours farre more rare
> These liquors sweet incorporated are ...
> Whales, Herons, bitours, strange oyles she makes
> With which dame natures errours she corrects,
> Using arts helpe to supply all defect (Knevet E3v–E4r).

In this standard, if unusually material, condemnation of vanity's artifice, Clematis interestingly draws upon the vocabulary of correctional imprisonment also found in the sonnets ('imprison', 'liquid prisoner'). Both texts evoke the image of a natural object trapped and transformed in the space of the home. And in identifying the household closet as the site in which art supplements nature, she echoes the most positively valued claims made by writers such as Plat. If artificial tampering usually indicates a problematic female agency in literary texts, recipe books render such supplementation necessary and virtuous.

Homework

Diaries and recipe books provide ample evidence that women, including elite ladies, did distill as part of kitchen work. As she made puddings, mutton, marmalade, pies, preserves, cough syrups, fritters, pancakes, leaches, salads, custards, breads, cakes, and sugar candy, Lady Elinor Fettiplace treated roses in stoppered bottles in her distillatory. Her recipe for oil of roses takes 12 months to make; her distilled strawberry water was used to heal 'the stone', to make almond puddings, and to create rosewater pancakes (Fettiplace 123). Similarly a miscellany composed between 1665 and 1822 indicates that at Bocker estate, Alice Bankes (Lady Borlase) oversaw cooking, baking, confectionary, and distillation. Her 'Way to distill Roses in Winter' maps an intricate process by which roses are layered with bay salt in earthen vessels and then buried underground for half a year before being distilled (Borlase 76).

Among the scrawled advice in Mary Granville's manuscript book, including 'To make one sleep', 'For a sore breast', 'To boil a haunch of venison', 'To Make an Admirable good water against Melancholy', 'To preserve walnuts', 'To cleane teeth well', and 'To Make a cake Mrs Margaret Melbourns Way', is one recipe entitled 'The manner of distilling water of honey'. This recipe advises the housewife to heat and cool white honey six or seven times in a glass still, watching its colour change from 'bloud' to 'Rubie' to 'gold'. Granville writes, in vivid terms, that it will

> be like to the coulor of gold, which then is most pleasant of savor and soe sweet that nothing may be compared like to it in fragrantness of smell. It doth dissolve gold and prepareth it to drinke. It is also very comfortable to all there that are apt to have swounding fitts, and are used to faintings in the stomacke – in giving to any one two or 3 drams to drinke. Likewise if you wash any wound or stripe with this water, it doth in small time heale the same; this pretious water doth marvelouely helpe the cough, the Rheume, the decease of the spleene and many other deseases scarce to be believed; This water was administred to a person sicke of the palsie for the space of 46 daies, and he was, by the mightie help of god and this miraculous water, thoroughly healed of his disease. Also this helpeth the falling sickness and preserveth the body from putrifying, soe that by all these wee may learn that this is as it were a divine water from heaven, and sent from God to serve unto all ages (38–9).

In creating a 'miraculous' and 'pretious' cure for coughs, fainting, palsy, and epilepsy, the housewife becomes an intermediary who transmits to mortals a divine solution. As 'blood' red properties convert to a gold-like essence, the housewife seems to boast an almost alchemical and divine power that bleeds over to describe the very bodies ingesting her mutating substance. She can keep the body from 'putrifying' in this fantastically described transformation.

The fact that some distillation recipes called for animals to be purified and boiled made it easier for readers to imagine flesh as an entity in need of domestic process. Almost every recipe book includes the standard recipe for 'cockwater', a heavily spiced chicken soup made through distillation. One 1582 recipe, 'our sirrup of a Capon' claims to offer 'a restorative of greate virtue':

> it is able to sustain a sick person many days without taking any other meat, because it is of flesh and blood, for the flesh sustaineth the flesh, and the blood sustaineth the blood, and the order to make it is thus. Take a great fat Capon that is well fleshed, and pull it while it is alive, and take forth only the guts an the belly, and when he is dead, stamp it in a Mortar grossly, and put it in a distilling glass with twenty pound of good white wine.. Salt, and ..Sugar and.. Cinnamon, then distill. (Fioravanti 59)

Here the castrated cock is plucked and degutted to create a jellied, spiced, alcoholic, and sweet chicken soup. In meat-based distillations, newly slaughtered animals whose spirits have not yet dissipated become face creams to prevent aging or nurturing cullises (see Murrell 2; Markham 131; Partridge D2r; Dawson 48).

It was perhaps the proximity of butchery to physic that prompted early modern writers to represent distillation as a threat to the integrity of the human creature. In *Hamlet*, Horatio describes the night watchmen as 'distill'd / Almost to jelly with the act of fear' upon seeing the ghost of Hamlet Sr. (1.2.204–5). Lady Macbeth not only drugs Duncan's guards with a posset but also describes the effects of her potion as a demonic housewifery. The two chamberlains, she plots, 'Will I with wine and wassail so convince, / That memory, the warder of the brain, / Shall be a fume, and the receipt of reason / A limbeck only' (1.7.64–7). Lady Macbeth seeks to turn the guards' brains into limbecks that vaporize rather than preserving their faculties of memory and reason. The source and the effect of her action collapse, as the body becomes a distillatory destructively imitating the substance it has ingested. Describing reason as a glass bottle turning memory into a fume, Lady Macbeth figures the early modern body's operations as kitchen work just at the moment that she is contemplating making a deadly posset, a household drink commonly found in recipe books.

In Shakespeare's most domestic play, *The Merry Wives of Windsor*, the famed Falstaff worries that he is distilled not by demons but by powerful housewives. After being dumped from a laundry basket stuffed with putrid clothes into a river, he offers a tirade that conflates his physical instability and sexual shame with daily household processes:

> To be stopp'd in like a strong distillation with stinking clothes that fretted in their own grease. Think of that – a man of my kidney. Think of that – that am as subject to heat as butter; a man of continual dissolution and thaw. It was a miracle to 'scape suffocation. And in the height of this bath (when I was more than half stew'd in grease, like a Dutch dish) to be thrown into the Thames, and cool'd, glowing hot, in that surge ... think of that. (3.5.112–22)

Falstaff's worry about being stewed, bathed and distilled is grounded in his acute awareness of the instability of humoral bodies in general but particularly his own vulnerability. His fantasy of liquefaction is highly domestic: the actual laundry basket mutates figuratively into a dairy cask, bathtub, cook pot, and limbeck. Rather than celebrating its ability to secure and preserve an essence, Falstaff sees distillation's alternate heating and cooling as ominously holding the power to evaporate the core of his overly humoral being. He identifies explicitly with the 'remainder' in distillation rather than the preserved product – the rose or metal altered when heated and cooled into a purified 'spirit'. As in many other literary works, distillation surfaces figuratively when characters express anxiety about lack of somatic control.

Artificial Souls

Restoring the domestic context of distillation to a reading of Shakespeare's early sonnets refines our understanding about the process of immortalization they describe. Seeing distillation in this light complicates the already complicated gendering of the 'procreation' recommended in this first group of poems.

Although everything is ambiguous in the *Sonnets*, the first group generally seems to be written by a male speaker who unusually advances reproduction as an option for combating his male beloved's mortality. While the speaker conventionally urges the beloved to seize the day, he atypically recommends sex with someone other than the speaker. In part because of these innovations, Shakespeare's *Sonnets* have surfaced in a body of criticism devoted to the history of gender and of sexuality.

Richard Halpern and Jeffrey Masten debate precisely how the trope of distillation, as articulated in Shakespeare's early sonnets, figure in these histories. Halpern argues that Shakespeare's *Sonnets* express an idealized form of desire, with Sonnet 5 offering a material (and aestheticized) 'treatise on poetic sublimation' (11). Halpern eloquently points out that while the metaphor of the perfume bottle

> bolsters the poem's longing for a beauty that transcends death, it fits somewhat
> awkwardly with its supposed tenor. In the translation from a child, to semen in
> a womb, to perfume in a bottle, something has been lost, and that something
> is life ... But if the image of perfume and glass is vastly ill-suited to its stated
> purpose of figuring sexual procreation, it is, as more than one critic has noticed,
> perfectly suited to another, implied purpose: that of figuring *poetic* procreation.
> The diminutive, unchanging perfection of the perfume bottle thus represents not
> a baby but a sonnet (9–10).

In the 'male womb of Shakespearean verse', a living being can persist past the point of death (10). Halpern goes on to note that while this substitution is not novel, it is proleptic, for it offers a 'curiously material demonstration, even before the fact, of the Freudian thesis that sexual desire can be sublimated into art' (11).

In response to Halpern's essay, Jeffrey Masten argues against equating distillation with sublimation. He instead advocates a more historicized reading of early modern rhetorics around procreation and distillation, one that recognizes that aesthetics and sexuality were entangled so thoroughly that one could not simply substitute for the other. Detaching the lofty meanings of the sublime, with its modern tie to sublimation, from distillation Masten notes that '*distill* ('to drip or trickle down' [*OED*]) and *sublime* (to 'set on high, lift vp', according to a 1604 hard-word list) are etymological opposites' (2). He then points out that seeing Sonnet 5's 'figuration of reproduction and poetry-writing more precisely as 'distillation' may ... remind us that 'procreation' in these sonnets is more about 'storage' than about creating something new ... I would thus describe the procreation sonnets as *re*creation sonnets: poems about men storing more men (in flesh of sons that recapitulate, print, or mirror fathers, *and* in words/poems)' (2). The young man is urged to treasure a vial, to locate in some 'no-place' the semen that will store men for the future.

Reading the *Sonnets* in this historicised discourse of distillation rather than in terms of an alchemical perfume alters the nature of the 'creation' that the first sonnets envision while putting pressure on 'the sublime' that sublimation supposedly produces. Imagining the beloved's act as something that early modern people associated with housewifery – indeed imagining the friend as a housewife performing insemination – disturbs the reproduction of male aristocratic fairness that the speaker urges. Whether distillation is sublimation or substitution (as Halpern and Masten debate), it pointedly locates an artificial production within the home, and thus the male-male dynamic by which babies and poems replicate is pressured by a discourse differently gendered than the critically noted metaphors of husbandry and tillage that pervade the early sonnets. If the female in the sexual triangle is relegated to the position of the limbeck, that designation is offset in part or complicated by the fact that the inseminator must play a role typically assigned to the housewife.[5]

Of course, the beloved is not just the distiller in Shakespeare's sonnet but also the rose distilled, the thing of beauty that is in need of preservation. It is in this collapse of agent and object that we glimpse a second confusion of gender categories. Tusser's account of the housewife 'plying' helps us to recognize the powerful domestic agency associated with distillation and other housewifely tasks that involved maintaining and manipulating people's bodies. As such, reference to the rose distiller might trail the structures of dependency fundamental to household life. Reliant upon the ministrations of housewives and their servants, early modern people sometimes described household tasks as requiring their awkward submission to bodily transformations (Wall 163–76). The domestic context of distillation thus might unlock in part the anxiety shadowing the proclamation of eternizing power in Sonnet 5. Why is the liberated rose – freed from time's grip – a 'prisoner', something, as Masten notes, necessarily pent up when penned, or written (4)? Why would the process of being rendered 'sweet' require the destruction of physical form? Does the self alter when reconfigured in the name of beauty? art? healthcare? or when reproduced in sonnets or books?

Let me return for a moment to Halpern, who, in a throw-away line, hints at how the complexities of distillation's everyday context dovetail with the poems' unusual representations of sexual reproduction. 'Somehow the sonneteers' rhetoric of seduction has gotten twisted in the direction of family values', Halpern writes, 'Indeed, the sense of imminent demise that pervades the poem works less to whip up a desperate sexual longing than to mortify desire into something merely prudent. It makes sex seem as exciting as putting up preserves' (8). Halpern's point is a good one; the physical act of sex described in Sonnets 5 and 6 does seem dryly functional – something drained of erotic energy and made to serve a larger social and aesthetic duty. Yet literary representations that I have examined elsewhere suggest that household tasks such as putting up preserves could be imagined in highly erotic ways in the period (Wall 51–3). Halpern's self-canceling simile momentarily unearths a domestic discourse in which function and pleasure are unusually intertwined.

Understanding distillation as a profoundly domestic activity does not simply aid our ability to refine the literary analysis of canonical works. An identification

---

[5]   One of Shakespeare's later sonnets, number 143, compares the speaker to the seemingly 'careful' but actually careless housewife who chases after chickens and forgets about her baby. While 'play[ing] the mother's part' is recognized by critics as part of the unexpected gender bending of these poems, the *Sonnets* might have engaged in this topic earlier when the speaker referenced domestic distillation.

of the everydayness of the trope figuring the immortalizing power of poetry can be imported back into a reading of the potential philosophical meanings of early modern everyday practice, the trace of which remain in prescriptive books. Although such a project extends beyond my scope, the recipe books of the period offer material that could lay the groundwork for seeing changes in the scientific definitions of experimentation and experience in the seventeenth century (Spiller). They also might illuminate the cognitive conundrums and meditations about art and nature raised in and through housework, the space for philosophical reflection that Primo Levi glimpsed as the possible beauty of distillation. The dedicatory address to one of Plat's recipe books, *The Jewell House of Art and Nature*, indicates that household experiments of many sorts might activate the type of searching contemplation raised in alchemical tracts and literary works. 'Although Nature appears a most fair and fruitful Body', D.B. states, 'yet the Art, here mentioned, is as a Soul to inform that Body to examine and refine her actions and to teach her to understand those abilities of her own, which before lay undiscovered to her' (*Jewell House* A2v). In fantasies of transformation, in which people are the agent and object of household practices, and nature informed by a kitchen-induced soul, we glimpse the knotty and gendered implications of matter in and of form, the inextricability of show and substance, the matter of art itself.

Works Cited

Anon. 1608. *A Closet for Ladies and Gentlewomen*. London. [H. Ballard] for Arthur Johnson.

———. 1655. *The Ladies Cabinet Opened and Enlarged*. London. T.M. for G. Bedell and T. Collins.

Bacon, Roger. 1597. *The Mirror of Alchimy*. London. [Thomas Creede] for Richard Olive.

Best, Michael. 1986. Ed. and Intro. Gervase Markam. *The English Housewife*. Kingston. McGill-Queen's University Press.

Borlase, Lady (Alice Banks). 1998. *Ladie Borlase's Receiptes Booke*. Ed. David E. Schoonover. Iowa City. University of Iowa Press.

Brunschwig, Hieronymus. 1527. *The vertuose boke of distyllacyon of the waters of all maner of herbes*. London. Laurens Andrewe.

Dawson, Thomas. 1587. *The good huswifes Jewell. Wherein is to be found most excellent and rare Devises for Conceites in Cookerie ... Whereunto is adjoined sundry approved receits for ... the way to distill many precious waters*. London. John Wolfe for Edward White.

Fettiplace, Elinor. 1986. *Elinor Fettiplace's Receipt Book: Elizabethan Country House Cooking*. Ed. Hilary Spurling. New York. Elisaeth Sifton Books Viking.

Fioravanti, Leonardo. 1582. *A Compendium of the rationall Secretes of ... Leonardo Phioravante Bolognese*. Trans. J. Hester. London. Jhon Kyngston, for George Pen, and J[ohn] H[ester].

Fleming, Juliet. 2001. *Graffiti and the Writing Arts of Early Modern England*. Philadelphia. University of Pennsylvania Press.

Gesner, Konrad. 1576. *The newe Jewell of health*. London. Henrie Denham.

Granville, Anne. c. 1640–1750. *Receipt Book*. Folger Library. V.a 430.

Greene, Thomas M. 1985. 'Pitiful Thrivers: Failed Husbandry in the Sonnets'. *Literary Theory/Renaissance Texts. Shakespeare and the Question of Theory*. Ed. Patricia Parker and Geoffrey Hartmann. New York. Methuen. 230–44.

Hall, Kim F. 1996. 'Culinary Spaces, Colonial Spaces: The Gendering of Sugar in the Seventeenth Century'. *Feminist Readings of Early Modern Culture: Emerging Subjects*. Ed. Valerie Traub, Lindsay Kaplan, and Dympna Callaghan. Cambridge: Cambridge University Press.

Halpern, Richard. 2001. 'Shakespeare's Perfume'. *Early Modern Culture: An Electronic Seminar. Issue 2*. http://emc.eserver.org/1–2/halpern.html.

Knevet, Ralph. 1631. *Rhodon and Iris*. London. John Beale for Michael Sparke.

Levi, Primo. 1984. *The Periodic Table*. Trans. Raymond Rosenthal. New York. Schocken Books.

Markham, Gervase. 1615. *The English Huswife. Country Contentments*. London. John Beale for R. Jackson.

Masten, Jeffrey. 2001. 'Gee, Your Heir Smells Terrific: Response to "Shakespeare's Perfume"'. *Early Modern Culture: An Electronic Seminar. Issue 2*. http://emc.eserver.org/1–2/masten.html.

Moran, Bruce, T. 2005. *Distilling Knowledge: Alchemy, Chemistry, and the Scientific Revolution*. Cambridge, MA. Harvard University Press.

Murrell, John. 1615. *New Book of Cookerie*. London. Printed for John Browne.

Newman, William. R. 2004. *Promethan Ambitions: Alchemy and the Quest to Perfect Nature*. Chicago, IL. University of Chicago Press.

Partridge, John. 1600. *A Treasurie of Commodious Conceits*. London. I. R[oberts] for Edward White.

Plat, Hugh. 1602. *Delights for Ladies*. London. Printed by Peter Short.

_____. 1653. *The Jewell House of Art and Nature*. London. Printed by Bernard Alsop.

Shakespeare, William. 1974. *The Riverside Shakespeare*. Ed. G. Blakemore Evans. Boston, MA: Houghton Mifflin.

Smith, Pamela. 2004. *The Body of the Artisan: Art and Experience in the Scientific Revolution*. Chicago, IL: University of Chicago Press.

Spiller, Elizabeth. 2008. 'Introduction'. *Seventeenth-Century English Recipe Books: Cooking, Physic and Chirurgery in the Works of Elizabeth Talbot Grey and Aletheia Talbot Howard*. Vol 3. *The Early Modern Englishwoman: A Facsimile Library of Essential Works*. Gen eds. Betty S. Travitsky and Anne Lake Prescott. Aldershot. Ashgate.

Tusser, Thomas. 1585. *Five Hundred Points of Good Husbandry*. London. Printed in the house of Henrie Denham.

Wall, Wendy. 2002. *Staging Domesticity: Household Work and National Identity in Early Modern England*. Cambridge: Cambridge University Press.

Woolley, Hannah. 1675. *The Queene-like Closet or Rich Cabinet*. London. Printed for Richard Lowndes.

PART 3
Food and Feeding in
Early Modern Literature

Chapter 6
Performances of the Banquet Course in Early Modern Drama

Tracy Thong

The sixteenth- and seventeenth-century banquet course was the early modern forerunner of our present-day dessert. Although much scholarly work relating to the historical and cultural significance of food and banqueting in the Renaissance has been written in the last decade or so, none of these has focused exclusively on the banquet course and how its language features in the drama of the period 1590–1640. Two of these works, Ken Albala's *The Banquet* and Joan Fitzpatrick's *Food in Shakespeare* were published in 2007, while others which have recently combined a culinary perspective with traditional literary analysis are *Aguecheek's Beef, Belch's Hiccup and Other Gastronomic Interjections*, *The Fury of Men's Gullets*, and *Banquets Set Forth* (Appelbaum 2006; Boehrer 1997; Meads 2001). Although all the works mentioned here have both informed and refined my research on the representation of dining rituals on the early modern stage, this essay will narrow the scope of Albala and Meads's studies on banqueting to focus specifically on the banquet course.

The clearest account of the evolution of the banquet course from the medieval to Renaissance periods, including its food, rituals, and setting of which it consisted, is provided in *'Banquetting Stuffe'* (Wilson, 1991). This collection contains a useful essay by Peter Brears, 'Rare Conceites and Strange Delightes', which includes recipes and illustrations of the sweets and biscuits that constituted sixteenth- and seventeenth-century banqueting fare (Brears 1991, 60–114). There are also several visual examples of the Continental banquet course that provide a valuable insight into the culinary trends being followed by the English. These sources include Clara Peeters's *Still-life* (1611), an oil on panel which shows wine goblets on a table, with a variety of nuts, crystallised confectionary, and knot-biscuits, or jumbles, on display. Another *Still-Life* (1610) by Floris Claesz Van Dijck shows fruit, nuts, wine, bread, and cheeses; in a bowl in the centre, are crystallised confections and biscuits such as biscuit-bread, knots, or jumbles, and letters. Another by Juan van der Hamen, a *Still-Life of Glass, Pottery, and Sweets* (1622), portrays what probably are hippocras and wafers, the main components of the medieval banquet, from which the early modern wine-and-sweetmeats course was derived.

As for the banquet setting, Coughton Court, in Warwickshire, has some very good examples of spaces used to accommodate both large feasts and dessert banquets. The property consists of a dining-room which was possibly the 'great chamber of the sixteenth-century house' (National Trust 2002, 14). This estate also has what is presently known as the 'tower room', an 'upper room [which] may have been used as a banqueting area, for sweet meats on special occasions after the main meal for the men only'. A spiral stairway from this room led to the roof, which, being flat, was conducive to guided walks for guests. It is also complete with a 'small shelter or study', which may have been used for intimate banquets or may have been where banqueting stuff was served while a larger number of guests milled around on the open rooftop (National Trust 2002, 12–13). These elevated spaces were also advantageous for impressing guests with outstanding views of the estate and surrounding countryside. Other features pertinent to this course include garden retreats, arbours, tree-houses, and buildings – such as orangeries, aviaries and menageries – to house unusual plants and animals for the admiration of guests.

One of the main distinguishing characteristics of the banquet course is the void, from which it first originated. Jennifer Stead discusses the specific rituals and proceedings that this entailed, as evolved from its medieval origins to its manifestations in the early modern period:

> The origins of the banquet are to be found in the medieval ending of a grand meal with hippocras and wafers, in the imported French ceremony of the *voidée* or void (which was additional wine and spices given after the tables had been cleared), and in the increasing use of sweetmeats, once considered medicinal and digestive – all coming together at the time of the early Tudors to make a separate final sweet course.

> The *voidée* is derived from the French *voider*, to clear the table, [or] to make empty, and so refers to the departure of guests and of those people leaving the Great Hall or Chamber who were not staying to sleep there; therefore the *voidée* refers to the final wine, spices, comfits, etc., taken before departing or retiring. [Sometimes,] while the servants eat, the company withdraws to another room and waits there till wine and spices are brought. [...] It is most likely that these are also consumed standing. [...] The practice of [which] may also be related to the practical points that tables had to be cleared and dismantled to allow for after-dinner activities such as games and dancing[.] (Stead 1991, 115)

The material accoutrements and the prospect afforded by the location of this withdrawing room contributed further to the recreations of the banquet course, and both also displayed the host's wealth.

Although commentaries relating to the banquet course traditionally occur in most plays of the period, the clearest depictions can be identified in well-known plays such as Shakespeare's *The Taming of the Shrew* (Shakespeare 1982), *Romeo and Juliet* (Shakespeare 2000), Middleton and Dekker's *The Roaring Girl* (Middleton and Dekker 1999), as well as Shakespeare and Middleton's relatively neglected *Timon of Athens* (Shakespeare and Middleton 2008) and Richard Brome's even less well-known *The Sparagus Garden* (Brome 1640). This essay will draw upon all the elements that constituted the main proceedings of the banquet course, and its identification of these rituals in the plays will be structured according to the traditional order of the proceedings. It will also look at the use of stage directions and dialogue to indicate the characters' mobility from the dining hall, where the principal meal is served, to the banqueting area, where wine and sweetmeats are being enjoyed with the accompanying rituals and amusements. It will determine the kind of banquet setting being staged – whether a withdrawing chamber or garden house, for example – and aims to evaluate these significations within the early modern domestic context.

According to John Jowett in his edition of *Timon of Athens* 'Shakespeare abandoned the play before it reached the stage', and the result is a 'starkly formal, simple and echoic' structure (Shakespeare and Middleton 2004, 1, 9); it is therefore appropriate that the rituals of standing on ceremony and the void are unusually prominent in *Timon of Athens* compared to the other plays considered here. Chris Meads has already recognised that Lucentio's banquet at the end of *The Taming of the Shrew* refers to the dessert course (Meads 2001, 100). The same observation applies to part of Lord Capulet's feast in *Romeo and Juliet* and Sir Alexander's banquet in the opening act of *The Roaring Girl*, the latter of which is an an irresistible example of how the formal rituals of the banquet course have been adapted for dramatic purposes. The subplot – which features citizens and their wives, gallants, and other city characters – also contains allusions to the banquet course when the Gallipots entertain their friends. In contrast, *The Sparagus Garden* is a uniquely different choice because its plot revolves around a location which supports and promotes the banquet course as a commercial enterprise.

Timon's first banquet in 1.2 of *Timon of Athens* is a prime example of the early modern ideal: 'a Liberal Entertainment of all sorts of Men, at one's House, whether Neighbours or Strangers, with kindness, especially with Meat, Drink, and Lodgings' (Heal 1990, 3). The accompanying stage direction certainly establishes his generosity: '*A great banquet served in*', but does not identify the type of banquet being presented here (1.2.1 s.d). John Jowett clarifies that this refers to 'a full banquet, as distinct from a light dessert […] the 'idle banquet' of l. 151' (Shakespeare and Middleton 2004, 189n). The indication that '*The* Lords *are standing with ceremony*' was an early addition by Samuel Johnson to clarify how the scene should be performed (1.2.14 s.d), and was probably justified by Timon's speech immediately after:

> Nay, my lords,
> Ceremony was but devised at first
> To set a gloss on faint deeds, hollow welcomes,
> Recanting goodness, sorry ere 'tis shown;
> But where there is true friendship, there needs none.
> Pray sit ... (1.2.13–18)

Timon's reference to 'ceremony' alludes to the ritual of voiding the tables, but, rather than showing them to a withdrawing room for the next course, he invites his guests to 'sit'. Both here and in *The Taming of the Shrew*, 'welcomes' are associated with the host expressly receiving a few guests to partake of the exclusive dessert banquet with him. However, Timon's opinion of these as 'hollow' is consistent with his indiscriminate reception of visitors up till now. In 1.1, he '*address*[*es*] *himself courteously to* every *suitor*' and refuses none of them: he agrees to pay Ventidius's debt, builds Lucilius's fortune so he may marry the old Athenian's daughter, promises to dine with everyone, including the poet, painter, and jeweller and excludes not even the cynical Apemantus or the unnamed 'Lords' from dinner (1.195 s.d; 1.1.259 s.d). But formal welcomes are crucial rituals of hospitality, since they allow the householder to maintain the exclusivity of their entertainment by distinguishing between 'those people leaving the Great Hall or Chamber who were not staying to sleep there' and those who were (Stead 1991, 115).[1] However, Timon callously disregards this economic necessity by receiving all his visitors to the '*great*' banquet and continues to receive 'certain nobles of the senate' even after the ladies have been 'dispose[d]' to the 'idle' banquet (1.2.1 s.d; 173; 151). These actions fit his dismissal of welcomes as 'hollow', and the movement of the plot towards his ruin.

The usual wine, nuts, and confections are mentioned in the other plays, but the fare served during Timon's great banquet is described as 'meat', 'blood', and 'bread' (1.2.38–47), implying that the meal is a grand feast rather than a banquet course. The descriptions also signify rather unusual exotica, since the meat, or food, on the table suggests Timon's flesh, as Shakespeare draws a comparison between Timon's banquet and the Last Supper. Apemantus also denounces Timon's guests for 'dip[ing] their meat in one man's blood' (1.2.41), followed by the Eucharistic undertones of this observation: 'The fellow that sits next him, now parts bread with him, pledges the breath of him in a divided draught, is the readiest man to kill him' (1.2.45–8). Thus, as Jowett's gloss indicates, the banquet course occurs only once the ritual of standing on ceremony is repeated: 'The Lords rise from table, with much adoring of Timon; and, to show their loves, each single out an Amazon, and all dance, men with women, a lofty strain or two to the oboes; and cease' (1.2.141 s.d). This rising marks the void, leading to a banquet course that is not fully enacted – the 'idle banquet' which is imagined offstage later in this scene (1.2.151). Jowett also observes:

> Such a dessert banquet might be offered to guests after an entertainment, but here it is offered only to the entertainers, getting the women immediately off stage. (Shakespeare and Middleton 2004, 201n)

In order to engineer this transition between meals, a masquer dressed as Cupid prompts the lords, having eaten, to rise from their table:

---

[1]   Although this implies that distinctions were made between guests 'staying' and those not, Stead is unclear about whether the distinctions lie between those sleeping in the Great Hall and those allocated a private chamber, or between guests staying on the host's premises, and those returning home. Either way, visitors who are given private chambers would be more highly regarded than those in a shared space, as are guests who are welcome to stay for an extended period versus those who are not.

Hail to thee, worthy Timon, and to all that of his bounties taste! The five best senses acknowledge thee their patron, and come freely to gratulate thy plenteous bosom.
There taste, touch, all, pleased from thy table rise,
They only now come but to feast thine eyes. (1.2.121–6)

Cupid's reference to the 'senses', especially sight, alludes to the display and spectacle which were central to the banquet course, because, after the 'rich and heavy meal' preceding this, 'diners would no longer be hungry, and so the nature of the banquet was not to satisfy the stomach, but to delight the eye' (Stead 1991, 120). His references to 'bounties', 'freely', and 'plenteous' also reiterate the ideal of liberality to impress guests with the abundance of Timon's resources to furnish his tables during entertainments. However, for the sake of household economy, it is only the projection of liberality which helps to secure the host's reputation, and not his practical adherence to this ideal. As with the first course, Timon is over-liberal with his hospitality: 'They're welcome all' (1.2.127).

In contrast to Sir Alexander, who takes the opportunity to show off his portraits, tapestries, and furniture during the transition from dining hall to withdrawing room in *The Roaring Girl* (Middleton and Dekker 1999, 1.2.1–32), Timon's dispensation of jewels and expensive gifts emphasizes his lavishness. Jewels, which feature prominently in this scene, could be incorporated in the banquet setting to imitate the jewel-like confections in an economical manner: 'Robert Laneham [...] describes the magnificent new aviary (probably used as a banqueting house) as being "a cage sumptuous and beautiful" [...] with columns, painted to look as if covered with diamonds, rubies, sapphires, and gold' (Stead 1991, 124). This description suggests that wealth and sumptuousness were manifest throughout the banquet, but not necessarily materialised, in order to boost the host's reputation. When Timon orders 'Lights, more lights!' and declares that he is 'Ready for his friends', this ensures that his galleries are in plain view as the lords exit. Thus, he needlessly gives the jewels and other items away to prove his status (1.2.235–8). And, whereas Sir Alexander leads his guests to a parlour where they may enjoy the prospect of his estate, Timon's generosity in giving out progressively larger gifts, from jewels and animals to his desire to part with 'lands' and the sum of his private 'kingdom' (1.2.225–30), is ultimately to the detriment of his honour and estate.[2]

In contrast to Timon's entertainment, the specificity with which guests are received applies to Lucentio's banquet course in 5.2 of *The Taming of the Shrew* as much as to hosts in the other plays. Its staging is clear when Lucentio announces: 'My banquet is to close our stomachs up / After our great good cheer' (5.2.9–10); this implies that small amounts of the expected wine and sweetmeats will now be consumed to aid digestion after their main meal. Shakespeare's presentation remains consistent with the traditional pattern of segregation between the location

---

2   Alexandra Shepard writes: 'If a man's worth was doubted, he lost his credit and was excluded from the relations of trust which both bound communities and accorded status and agency' (Shepard 2003, 193).

of the principal meal and dessert. In 5.1, Vincentio insists that Petruchio and his companions stay for some 'cheer' for showing him to Lucentio's house (5.1.12). Unfortunately, they are all excluded from entertainment on account of the elaborate disguise plot devised by the latter to court Bianca, but Lucentio eventually compensates for this by graciously receiving everyone to his banquet. In his book on table talk, Michel Jeanneret asserts, 'During a meal, conversation should erase differences, remove hierarchy and overcome inhibition [...] Always striking the right note and remaining "elegant, urbane and ingenious" is a subtle art' (Jeanneret 1991, 93). As his welcoming speech would suggest, Lucentio is a proficient and inclusive host who seeks to 'erase differences':

> At last, though long, our jarring notes agree,
> And time it is when raging war is done
> To smile at scapes and perils overblown.
> My fair Bianca, bid my father welcome,
> And I with selfsame kindness welcome thine.
> Brother Petruchio, sister Katherina,
> And thou, Hortensio, with thy loving widow,
> Feast with the best, and welcome to my house. (5.2.1–8)

Yet, considering the hierarchisation involved in first welcoming both fathers, then siblings and friends, and omitting mention of other guests entirely, even Lucentio's speech suggests that, in order to achieve the ideals pertaining to convivial discourse, tensions and other 'jarring notes' must be evident. This example shows that the early modern elite erased differences which posed a threat or challenge to the subsistence of their social group, and maintained their elegance, by restoring the social hierarchy. 'Differences' and 'hierarchy' are continually reasserted throughout this banquet course before the 'right note' is finally achieved. Petruchio provokes differences between himself and Hortensio by alleging that he 'fears his widow' for some after-dinner amusement (5.2.16). These, the widow erases by evoking Kate's shrewishness to align the pair together – 'He that is giddy thinks the world turns round' (5.2.20). The resulting competition between the widow and Kate is resolved when the men wager on their wives' obedience. Finally, their differences are erased once Petruchio proves that he is equal to other husbands for having imposed his authority over his wife, and for his desire to promote the virtues and worth of his household. Although it appears that virtually all the characters have been received to this banquet, Lucentio certainly does not include such nondescript characters as the tailor, haberdasher, or the jeweller, painter, poet, and unnamed lords whom Timon so enthusiastically entertains. Instead, the promising young householder prudently asserts: 'Feast with the *best*, and welcome to my house' (5.2.8; my italics).

The banquet course not only takes place in the final act of *The Taming of the Shrew* but is referred to extensively throughout, particularly when the lord arranges for his servingmen to bring 'A most delicious banquet by [Sly's] bed' and invite him to 'taste of [...] conserves' (Ind.1.36; Ind.2.3). As with *Timon of Athens* and *Romeo and Juliet*, Shakespeare uses structural elements to adapt the ritual of the void and the transition between rooms which accompanies it in these scenes. The lord's order that the huntsmen 'sup [the hounds] well, and look unto them all' immediately precedes his encounter with Sly and the latter's relocation to a chamber in the lord's house (Ind.1.25). The 1623 First Folio of Shakespeare gives no clear indication of where the induction scenes are set (Shakespeare 1968, 226–8) but the first induction scene probably takes place in front of the hostess's tavern, and the second, in which the wine and banqueting conceits are served to Sly, in the lord's 'fairest chamber' (Ind.1.43). Shakespeare distinguishes the banquet course from a principal, sustaining meal by contrasting wine with small ale, and sweet conserves with conserves of beef. Not only does the banquet course subvert Sly's ordinary expectations but also its order of proceedings is inverted from the norm: instead of wine and sweetmeats before bed, Sly is presented with the banquet when he awakes from his ale-induced stupor. This inversion of the conventional arrangement indicates how far the lord's banquet departs from Sly's daily circumstances. This experience serves as a stark reminder that for Sly, who was thrown out of a tavern for his lack of social credit, being entertained at such a banquet is 'a flattering dream or worthless fancy' (Ind.1.41).

In *Romeo and Juliet*, too, Lord Capulet is not so indiscriminate as to receive the entire Veronese community to his entertainment, but he proves himself to be an exemplary host nonetheless. He includes Paris in the numbers with this invitation:

> This night I hold an old-accustomed feast,
> Whereto I have invited many a guest,
> Such as I love; and you among the store,
> One more, most welcome, makes my number more. (1.2.20–23)

When his servingman approaches Romeo to help him read the guest list, it is clear that, unsurprisingly, the Montagues are not amongst those loved by Capulet: 'My master is the great rich Capulet, and if you be not of the house of Montagues, I pray come and crush a cup of wine' (1.2.81–3). Despite his family's exclusion, Romeo attends the feast disguised, hoping to meet Rosaline. But when Tybalt discovers his presence, Capulet stands firmly against any confrontation between them, enemy or not, on these grounds:

> A bears him like a portly gentleman,
> And, to say truth, Verona brags of him
> To be a virtuous and well-governed youth.
> I would not for the wealth of all this town
> Here in my house do him disparagement. (1.4.179–83)

Romeo and his friends approach Capulet's household tactically, as masquers, for, by the time they enter to partake of the evening's entertainment, 'Supper is done' (1.4.103). Mercutio's tale of Queen Mab also raises the audience's anticipation of the 'trifling foolish banquet towards' which Capulet promises his guests before they leave (1.4.235):

> Her chariot is an empty hazelnut
> […]
> And in this state she gallops night by night
> […]
> O'er ladies' lips, who straight on kisses dream,
> Which oft the angry Mab with blisters plagues
> Because their breaths with sweetmeats tainted are. (1.4.65–74)

Mercutio relentlessly teases the lovelorn Romeo by evoking the titillating promises of erotic stimuli associated with nibbling on sugary aphrodisiacs before retiring to bed. This is enhanced by the image of a wanton fairy who comes, galloping in a spent nutshell (Shakespeare 2000, 184n). Hazelnuts frequently appeared on banqueting tables, as shown in my earlier description of still-life paintings. In the scene before, a serving-man reports that 'the guests are come, supper served up' to prompt his mistress to attend to their companions (1.3.102–3). And, later, he and the other servants are bustling to clear the tables:

> <CHIEF> SERVING-MAN Where's Potpan, that he helps not to take away? He shift a trencher, he scrape a trencher!
> […]
> <CHIEF> SERVING-MAN   Away with the joint-stools, remove the court-cupboard, look to the plate. Good thou, save me a piece of marchpane, and as thou loves me, let the porter let in Susan Grindstone and Nell, Anthony and Potpan.
> SECOND SERVING-MAN Ay, boy, ready.
> <CHIEF> SERVING-MAN You are looked for and called for, asked for and sought for, in the great chamber.
> THIRD SERVING-MAN We cannot be here and there too. Cheerly, boys! Be brisk a while, and the longest liver take all. (1.4.113–28)

Shakespeare's portrayal of servants voiding the supper in this scene demonstrates his sympathy towards them, even when they claim a few perks on the job. The first serving-man enters one of the private rooms from the dining hall, 'with napkins' probably from the supper tables (1.4.112 s.d). Although he covets a piece of marzipan and looks forward to keeping company with Susan Grindstone – whose name also implies industry – and Nell, he works diligently to allow for Capulet's next course and objects when Potpan takes too many liberties by saving leftovers from all the trenchers for himself. There appears to be a further miscommunication between servants and master which hinders the process: the tables and chairs are set out for the banquet course by the time the Capulets, guests, and masquers enter, but Capulet then orders that the tables be turned up to make space for dancing.

Either way, when Tybalt identifies Romeo, the void has already taken place, thus depriving them of the suave exclusion of less favoured guests that this ceremony afforded its practitioners. This is not to say that once present, guests may be turned away partway through the entertainment, but the plays clearly demonstrate the means by which hosts could ensure that their prejudice against certain members of the party was still palpable. As mentioned previously, one of these means was the kind of welcome that the host extended to his guests. This observation applies equally to Capulet as to Lucentio. Since it occurs when the former invites his guests to dance, this example will be presented later in a combined discussion of after-dinner entertainment in Timon's masque of Amazons and the dancing ladies in *The Sparagus Garden*.

In *The Roaring Girl*, the quality of entertainment afforded by Sir Alexander's household is also based on prescribed conditions, namely, status and gender. The play's structuring of the void and ceremonial rising from tables is evident in the stage directions and dialogue of Act 1. The 1611 Quarto gives no consistent indication of acts or scenes in the play, but the segregation of plot and setting are sufficiently evident for editors to have indicated where such divisions are appropriate. The formality of rising after the main meal for the dining area to be voided, either for the servants' meal or for the rest of the evening's entertainment, is imagined offstage in 1.1, when Sebastian issues this instruction to Neatfoot: 'Prithee look in, for all the gentlemen are upon rising' (1.1.42). The party enters in 1.2, all thanking Sir Alexander for their 'bounteous cheer', and are shown to the parlour where he orders wine to be served, because, as he puts it: 'Th'inner room was too close' (1.2.1, 6), that is, to the rest of his household, affording them little privacy from the servants and other occupants. His enquiry of 'how do you like / This parlour, gentlemen?' is a coded signal for his guests to compliment what they see in his show of conspicuous consumption (1.2.7). Also, by the time Sebastian appears on stage 'his belly is replenished', for Neatfoot expresses a certain smug complacence at having 'culled out for him […] a daintier bit or modicum than any lay upon his trencher at dinner' when Mary Fitzallard seeks an audience with Sebastian, whereby 'a daintier bit' compares her to delicate banqueting conceits before retiring (1.1.10–12).

Middleton and Dekker continually emphasise their staging of the banquet course in this act by using the characters onstage to comment on the servants' activities offstage. While waiting for Sebastian to finish supper, Neatfoot invites Mary to join the servingmen 'in the hall […] and take such as they can set before [her]' from the available victuals, or 'kiss the lip of a cup of rich Orleans in the butt'ry amongst our waiting-women'. Most likely, the first refers to servants having their meal after the dining hall has been voided, while the women, like Mary, 'have dined […] already' and are having some after-dinner wine, which prefigures Sir Alexander's order for wine during his banquet (1.1.16–21).

This sequence successfully conveys the exclusivity of the dessert course with the playwrights' unconventional association of banqueting with servants, and through the portrayal of Sir Alexander's attitude towards his servants and guests. He withdraws to the parlour – a more exclusive and luxurious space suitable to accommodate 'a mess of friends' – and leaves the dining room to his servants (1.2.59). Mary is clearly not welcome to Sir Alexander's entertainment; neither, of course, are his servants, whom Neatfoot perceives to be of equivalent status to her. Sir Alexander further highlights the distinctions between his social group and servants by summoning them for service, addressing them as 'knaves', 'varlets', and accusing them of 'Kissing [his] maids, drinking, or [being] fast asleep' (1.2.42–5). Neatfoot admits to the last, and the allusions to wine and delicacies (maids to kiss) before retiring reinforces the banquet theme. Later in the scene, Trapdoor vows to be so fastidious in his service as 'To be a shifter under your worship's nose of a clean trencher, when there's good bit upon 't' (1.2.190– 91). While this expresses, with mock earnestness, that he is so anxious to please his new master that he will clear the table long before it is necessary, or indeed, desired, by Sir Alexander, it also acknowledges the divide between the Wengraves and their social lessers. The only means by which the less privileged may enjoy the exclusive pleasures afforded by the banquet course is, like the servingmen in *Romeo and Juliet*, to seize an opportunity when it arises. Unlike Sir Alexander and those of his class, the servants' position affords them time for pleasure and recreation only surreptitiously, because conspicuous consumption is a privilege not available to them.

Sir Alexander also manifests the exclusivity of his banquet by allocating chairs and stools according to each guest's importance. He assigns chairs to guests who are either superior or equal to himself: a 'back-friend' each is found for Sir Davy and Sir Adam (1.2.49), while Goshawk's response to the invitation to 'perch' with 'I stoop to your lure, sir', indicates the figurative parallels between low seating and low social status (1.2.52–3). Seating for Greenwit is left to Sebastian and unminded by Sir Alexander altogether; Laxton is mocked for 'want[ing] – a stone' to indicate that he is perceived as physically and socially impotent. He is then offered a stool and callously left to stand when he takes offence at the provocation (1.2.56). Considering that great significance was attached to a heightened prospect of views across his estate when a host wished to impress others, the guests who are not offered chairs are thus not afforded a 'privileged view of the house's bounty' (Richardson 2006, 77).

Although the setting of Brome's *Sparagus Garden* is not explicit, Matthew Steggle observes that it stands on 'seemingly reclaimed land in an unspecified South Bank marsh' – it is easily accessible to its urban clientele and is 'a rendezvous for the fashionable smart set'. The play presents an interesting adaptation of the banquet course because it supports early modern accusations of the banquet setting's ill repute and clearly reflects the extramarital liberties that asparagus gardens afforded their visitors. Steggle identifies Brome's garden as 'a potential location for sin and crime of various sorts' and argues compellingly that it was inspired by a real asparagus garden in London (Steggle 2004, 71–83). In order to attract customers to the play's garden, Sir Hugh Moneylacks advertises it as a place of luxury by punning on plant beds and beds (or couches) to sleep in and emphasising that it affords discretion for those who prefer to retire into the house:

> […] the house affords you as convenient Couches to retyre to, as the garden has beds for the precious plants to grow in: that makes the place a pallace of pleasure, and daily resorted and fill'ed with Lords and Knights, and their Ladies; Gentlemen and gallants with their Mistresses[.] (D1r–v)

Even though the business needs custom to maintain its profits, its proprieters nonetheless strive to maintain its exclusivity. This is evident in Brome's presentation of the void and the conflict which householders' weeding and classification of clients posed against the ideal that hosts entertained all guests liberally.

The Gardner's projection of liberality is demonstrated by the pleasure garden, where their own prized asparagus is grown and served with wine and sweetmeats for their guests' delectation. For, 'it was a matter of pride to one's self and it flattered one's friends if one offered them fare that was both attractive and *home-made*' (Wilson 1991, 30), such that, as a further example, 'a rare and delicate peach from one's own estate, carefully tended and matured to perfection, was often presented as tangible evidence of a landowner's pride of place and mastery over nature' (Albala 2007, 1). The asparagus garden is clearly a trope for the characters' aspirations towards upward mobility. Other than its proprieters, Gardner and his wife Martha, these aspirants include the Brittlewares, a couple trying to conceive; a gull named Hoyden, who believes that squandering his money on expensive food and drink will make him a gentleman; the errant knight Sir Hugh Moneylacks (referred to above), who entices them all to the asparagus garden; and three young men – Sam, Gilbert, and Walter – who must remain in their fathers' favour to inherit their family's wealth and status.

The void is not very distinct in this text, but it is plausible to argue that Brome has adapted it to Martha's refusal of a room at the garden's premises for Sam, Walter, and Gilbert. In 3.3, the trio seek to find a way – over some wine, sweetmeats, and asparagus – for Sam to marry Annabella without provoking his father's displeasure. In contrast to the distinctions between guests staying with their hosts and those not, all guests are, of course, welcome at the asparagus garden to keep the business running. However, those visiting with female companions are clearly accorded preferential status, for Martha claims that there are no rooms left for the three of them:

> GILBERT Did you note the wit o' the woman?
> WALTER I, because we had no wenches we must have no chamber-roome, for feare she disappoynt some that may bring them. (F1r)

The play takes its appropriation of the void at face value; Martha literally clears the trio out of the 'chamber-roome' by claiming that they are 'taken up' (F1r). Her excuse is similar to Capulet's instruction for his servants to 'turn the tables up' in *Romeo and Juliet* (1.4.140). Just as Martha reserves her rooms in anticipation of higher-spending customers, so Capulet intends his 'great chamber', presently furnished with tables and chairs, to be used for the masquers' dance after the main meal (1.4.125). Capulet too discriminates against his guests according to gender. While Martha shows Sam, Walter, and Gilbert out to the garden for lack of women amongst their company, Capulet enlists his female guests' assistance in providing entertainment by compelling them to dance with his male guests. The basis for his attitude will be discussed in tandem with Timon's masque of Amazons later in this essay.

Similar to Sir Alexander's strategic seating arrangements, Brome suggests that hosts imposed a kind of classification process upon their guests when undertaking hospitality. It was customary to stand or walk around while partaking of the banquet course, and it seems that this, together with the void, was often due to spatial constraints within the household. The dining hall was cleared 'to allow for after-dinner activities such as games and dancing, and in very large households the only place where large numbers of servants could sit down to eat was the Great Hall', so the void also facilitated servants' mealtimes (Stead 1991, 118). In consequence, the banquet course was, unlike the main feast, characterised by its mobility, although more distinguished guests could be offered less walking between dining hall and banqueting room on their full stomachs to enjoy the privilege of superior views of the estate. In *The Sparagus Garden*, lower status or credibility is certainly attached to walking around the garden rather than being assigned the privilege of a room from which the prospect can be enjoyed. The Gardners' reason for this discrimination is based on the general hypothesis that visiting couples appreciate a discreet place of assignation, and deserve it, since the men are likely to spend more to impress their female escorts. Their theory turns out to be accurate, as the profit made from the knight entertaining his lady-like escort is 'pretty well for two'. At the other end of the scale, her husband, who is obviously complicit in his 'broken' wife's intimacies with other men and positively encourages it for the couple's financial benefit, spends little while keeping an eye on her at the garden. He buys only one bottle of wine for each of his party and shares out a dish of asparagus and some cheap, 'broken [sweet]meate' amongst them. The other significant distinction being made here is that all the women accompanying the guests who are assigned bed chambers are married: 'the poore young gentlemans wife' and 'the broken citizens wife'. Another gentleman insinuates that Martha has performed the same function – 'I protest Mr. Gardner your wife is too deare' (E4r–v). The '1630s vision of an asparagus garden as a place that offers women, in particular, a sexual freedom outside marriage is something reflected in Brome's play' (Steggle 2004, 72). In contrast, the companionless Sir Arnold Cautious contents himself with 'walk[ing] about the garden here halfe a day together, to feed upon Ladyes looks, as they passe to and fro' (E4v), and the three gallants are extended a limited welcome to 'bestow [them]selves in the garden' (F1v).

In the plays under consideration, scenes that depict entertainment such as masques and dancing typified the recreations which accompanied the banquet course. This is highly stylised in *Timon of Athens*, with guests participating in the masque of Amazons by dancing with the ladies before men and women withdraw to the banquet course in separate rooms. Timon shows the ladies out of the dining hall with this invitation: 'there is an idle banquet attends you, / Please you to dispose yourselves' (1.2.154–5); that the repast is described as 'void of any real worth, value or significance' accurately reflects our modern perspective of the banquet course's nutritional value, while highlighting Timon's modesty.[3] It is possible that Timon's invitation to the ladies also bears the connotation that they should dispose themselves to the idle appetites of the male guests for erotic stimuli, after 'the final wine, spices, comfits, etc., taken before departing or retiring' (Stead 1991, 115). The association is emphasised further when Timon

---

[3]   *OED* ('idle' *a.*); Fumerton asserts that 'the essential food value of banqueting stuffs [...] was *nothing*' (Fumerton 1991, 133).

praises them for having 'added worth unto't and lustre, / And entertained me with mine own device' (1.2.148–9). This 'device' refers to his banquet, while 'worth' and 'lustre' simultaneously denote the high value of sugar in terms of its medicinal properties as well as its costliness.[4] Within the discourse of Timon's banquet, the ladies become inextricably linked to the sweetmeats consumed by the men before they depart or retire, with their presence substituting that of the banqueting stuff on stage. The entertainment derived by the lords from being paired with the ladies also adds worth to the event, in that, theoretically, it boosts Timon's social credit with those who have partaken of it.

Capulet, too, expects that the ladies at his banquet will add lustre to his entertainment and volunteers their company to his male guests when the dancing begins:

CAPULET
Welcome, gentlemen. Ladies that have their toes
Unplagued with corns will walk a bout with you.
Ah my mistresses, which of you all
Will now deny to dance? She that makes dainty,
She I'll swear hath corns. Am I come near ye now?
Welcome, gentlemen. I have seen the day
That I have worn a visor, and could tell
A whispering tale in a fair lady's ear,
Such as would please. 'Tis gone, 'tis gone, 'tis gone.
You are welcome, gentlemen. Come, musicians, play.
Music plays and they dance
A hall, a hall! Give room, and foot it, girls. –
More light, you knaves, and turn the tables up,
And quench the fire, the room is grown too hot. –
Ah sirrah, this unlooked-for sport comes well. –
Nay sit, nay sit, good cousin Capulet,
For you and I are past our dancing days. (1.4.129–44)

It is unclear if 'Give room' is an instruction for the ladies to make way for the menfolk, as the punctuation in this edition suggests, or whether it is directed to the servants who should clear the tables away to make more space. His instruction for the fire to be quenched acts as further indication of the emphasis on male pleasure during rituals and pastimes associated with the void. Men were perceived as hot and dry in constitution according to early modern humoral theory, so the necessity that the fire needs putting out suggests that the testosterone-charged atmosphere of men being entertained by the dancing girls should be countered by elements that are cold and moist. Water presumably fulfils this need and symbolises the female constitution, but it is worth noting that, unlike the fire, this element goes unmentioned. Capulet's reference to the ladies 'making dainty' is, of course, a

---

4   Fumerton writes: 'So valuable and rare were spiced sugars […] that they were locked away in cabinets as if they were jewels. Indeed, confectionery and sweetmeats were often compared to jewels' (Fumerton 1991, 134).

common pun on banqueting dainties, or delicacies, and alludes to the female task of making the sugar-based fare for the banquet course. Similar to Sir Alexander's treatment of his guests in *The Roaring Girl*, sitting is regarded as the position of privilege and seniority.

The last play of this selection which features dancing as an accompaniment to the banquet course is *The Sparagus Garden*. In 3.6, a pair of courtiers invite ladies to dance with them in the Gardner's knot garden:

1 COURTIER Come Madams, now if you please after your garden Feast,
To exercise your numerous feet, and tread
A curious knot upon this grassie square;
You shall fresh vigour adde unto the spring,
And double the encrease, sweetnesse and beauty
Of every plant and flower throughout the garden.
1 LADY If I thought so my Lord, we would not doe
Such precious worke for nothing; we would be
Much better huswifes, and compound for shares
O'th' gardners profit.
2 LADY Or at least hedge in
Our Sparagus dinner reckoning.
2 COURTIER I commend your worldly providence:
Madam, such good Ladies will never dance
Away their husbands Lands.
1 COURTIER But Madams will yee dance?
1 LADY Not to improve the garden good my Lord,
A little for digestion if you please. (F4r–v)

Unlike the ladies in Shakespeare's *Timon of Athens* and *Romeo and Juliet*, Brome gives his ladies a voice. Although any offence caused by the first courtier's invitation may be unwitting, as he seeks to clarify his request in 'But Madams will yee dance?', it could be construed as an attempt to mix pleasure with work, since it links the garden which has been designed for the pleasure of the Gardners' clientele with women's work (F4v), in particular, Martha's 'helping hand […] and braine […] in the businesse' (E4r).

Paula Henderson makes the observation that aspects of horticultural landscaping, in particular knot gardens, were attributed to the lady of the household:

In *The Country House-wifes Garden* Markham published nine complex designs for knots and one for the maze, beginning with a simple 'ground plot for knots' that showed the reader how to begin by squaring up her garden. This he saw as simply a guide, however, lest he deprive the housewife of the joys of experimenting with her own designs, […] demonstrating how personal these gardens were. (Henderson 2005, 122)[5]

---

[5]   *The Country House-wifes Garden*, though often attributed to Markham, was actually written by Willam Lawson. See Lawson 1618.

If knot-garden designs were really unique to the mistress of the household, then the ladies' treading of knots in the garden as they wear out the turf with their dancing represents an encroachment upon Martha's self-expression and autonomy in her duties.

Such an encroachment upon Martha's work would have been intensely personal. The lady's reference to 'huswifes', or hussies, also emphasizes the delicate balance between women labouring with their bodies for the benefit of their household and that which is detrimental to their social esteem and the reputation of their estate. Hence the ladies refuse to 'worke for nothing'; neither do they 'compound for shares / O'th' gardners profit' (F4v). Instead, their agreement to dance 'A little for digestion' defines them as well-mannered guests who, as Gilbert anticipates earlier in the play, are 'noble ones, the three Graces of the Court, the Lady Stately, the Lady Handsome, and the Lady peerelesse' (F2r; Steggle 2004, 82–3; Hamilton 1990, 'Graces').[6]

The reference to knots pertains not only to the housewife's tasks in the garden, because its replication in the form of knot biscuits, which Markham calls 'jumbles', further exemplifies the fusing of skill, taste, and intellect which is so fundamental to the banquet course (Best 1986; Markham 1986, ii/ 156, 158; Brears 1991, 89, 97–8). Once more, his reader is encouraged to 'make them in what forms you please', thus identifying another product used to display the individuality of its creator (Best 1986; Markham 1986, ii/ 156). Hence, as knot gardens and knot biscuits form intrinsic components to banqueting display, the courtiers' invitation to their female companions in the above extract might result in the treading of toes rather than knots, thus undermining the basis of kind and liberal hospitality, which is reciprocity. The first lady's diplomatic agreement to dance, but on the firm condition that she will do so 'for digestion', and 'not to improve the garden', emphasizes the healthful benefits of the banquet course. It also asserts the women's determination to partake in the pleasures of the garden and not to intrude on the activities which go towards maintaining its setting, to engage in promiscuous behaviour like 'the broken citizens wife' (E4r), nor to increase 'the gardners profit' by 'add[ing] worth' to their entertainment (*Timon*: 1.2.145).

Although this essay covers all formal banqueting rituals, it is impossible to do justice to the full range of variations which occur in early modern plays. Since banquets were elite occasions and highly regarded, their accompanying rituals were emulated by hosts and guests of all classes and conditions. This examination is based on the assumption that performances of the banquet course, whether on stage or in early modern households, were more likely to adapt the rigours of tradition and ideals than conform to them. The same approach to the variety of recreations that could accompany the banquet course has also been taken here. Although dancing is most pervasive, being common to three of the plays discussed,

---

[6]   Steggle comes to a similar conclusion as Hamilton by emphasising that 'the solidity of land […] on which they dance' reflects 'the continuing prosperity and fertility of the Sparagus Garden' (Steggle 2004, 82–3).

other entertainments also occur in these texts. These include games or gambling, such as the wager on wives' obedience in *The Taming of the Shrew* which was briefly discussed; Petruchio also refers rather grandiosely to forms of entertainment he has witnessed:

> Have I not in my time heard lions roar?
> Have I not heard the sea, puffed up with winds,
> Rage like an angry boar chafed with sweat?
> Have I not heard great ordnance in the field,
> And heaven's artillery thunder in the skies?
> Have I not in a pitched battle heard
> Loud 'larums, neighing steeds, and trumpets' clang? (1.2.196–202)

My assumption about the modes of entertainment available to Petruchio is supported when he uses Kate to substitute for a fountain display during Lucentio's banquet at the end of 5.2. On this occasion, Kate dutifully informs Bianca, the widow, and everyone present that 'A woman moved is like a fountain troubled / Muddy, ill-seeming, thick, bereft of beauty' (5.2.146–7). Kate's public demonstration of her obedience to Petruchio during Lucentio's entertainment proves that she is no longer 'troubled' but looked upon with 'wonder' and admired, like a banquet display, by all the guests (5.2.193). This expectation is maintained throughout the play by Petruchio's persistent punning on Kate and 'cate', particularly in this instance:

> But Kate, the prettiest Kate in Christendom,
> Kate of Kate Hall, my super-dainty Kate,
> For dainties are all Kates ... (2.1.185–7)

Having finally tamed her, Kate makes a fine 'cate' or delicacy, specially moulded for display and now plashes not water, but advice to other women on marital conduct.

In the induction, the lord's servingmen offer Sly entertainment which is supported by the estate – such as a gallery of erotic paintings, riding, hawking, and hunting – when the latter remains unimpressed with the fruit or flower conserves, and unconvinced about his 'lady' (Ind. 2.24). Their improvisation produces wonderful comedy, for, when Sly starts to believe the fabrication: 'Am I a lord, and have I such a lady?' (Ind. 2.66), he bids the cross-dressed Bartholomew to 'undress [...] and come now to bed' (Ind. 2.115).

When Timon becomes destitute, he takes the form of a wildman and seeks refuge in the woods outside Athens. Shakespeare's reference here alludes to forested areas on large estates which were used by householders to simulate real wildernesses and a variety of stock imaginary characters lurking within, such as savage men, the Lady of the Lake, nymphs, wild beasts, and singing bushes, especially during royal entertainments. In 4.3, Alcibiades and the whores demand that the wild Timon identifies himself when they wander into the woods and the latter maintains his persona like the masquer playing Cupid; he presents them with gifts in a manner in keeping with the wildman by throwing gold at them. Shakespeare's use of forests and wildernesses as a trope for the banquet setting occurs quite extensively in his plays, with other examples including *As You Like It*, *The Tempest*, *Titus Andronicus*, and *The Winter's Tale*. Brome's asparagus garden, though a natural setting too, is rather more benign than Shakespeare's versions, with carefully weeded plant beds, knot gardens and shady arbours. However, its purpose is similar to Timon's woods in that the garden is frequented by city dwellers who wish to seek refuge away from the prying eyes of the public.

Other recreations associated with the banquet course include smoking. Middleton and Dekker establish tobacco-smoking as a substitute for the delicacies usually savoured during banquets through the tightly structured sequence of their opening act. Sir Alexander's banquet in 1.2, and Neatfoot's references to the servants' surreptitious emulation of this throughout the act, is followed by a street scene that features Laxton, Greenwit, and other gallants savouring the '[p]ure and excellent' qualities of Mrs Gallipot's tobacco rather vociferously, such that their desire to be seen and heard partaking of this 'banquet' is apparent (2.1.54).

Although the historical banquet course could be set in a wide variety of locations, the conditions of settings are quite similar in these plays. Sir Alexander has his banquet course in an elevated parlour which holds six. It is possible that Middleton and Dekker imagined the architectural layout of his lodgings as one similar to the surviving example at Coughton Court, perhaps with subtle variations in size. In contrast, Timon and Lord Capulet's banqueting halls are large enough to accommodate dances involving their entire local community or, perhaps, in Capulet's case, members of his Veronese peer group. Timon's household, similar to Lucentio's, contains at least one additional chamber which withdraws from the main dining hall. It is where the women retire, for the 'idle' banquet, in Timon's case (1.2.151). Had the Gallipots' banquet come to fruition, this would probably have taken place in a room on the ground or first floor, since mercantile properties generally consisted of two levels, and probably some loft space. It is difficult to tell with *The Sparagus Garden*, but space for customers who wish to banquet is available in outdoor arbours as well as rooms within. Since the Gardners rent the land they cultivate, it is possible that the latter takes the form of ground or first floor lodgings too. Once more, this selection of plays does not account for the full range of settings in which the early modern banquet course took place; however, these dramatic examples reflect a lived reality in which level of income and social background posed no barrier against people of different conditions seeking to emulate aristocratic dining rituals as far as their means allowed.

Works Cited

Albala, Ken. 2002. *Eating Right in the Renaissance*. California Studies in Food and Culture, 2. Berkeley. University of California Press.

———. 2007. *The Banquet: Dining in the Great Courts of Late Renaissance Europe*. Urbana and Chicago. University of Illinois Press.

Appelbaum, Robert. 2006. *Aguecheek's Beef, Belch's Hiccup, and other Gastronomic Interjections: Literature, Culture and Food Among the Early Moderns*. Chicago, IL.University of Chicago Press.

Boehrer, Bruce. T. 1997. *The Fury of Men's Gullets: Ben Jonson and the Digestive Canal*. Philadelphia. University of Pennsylvania Press.

Brears, Peter. 1991. 'Rare Conceites and Strange Delights'. In *'Banquetting Stuffe': The Fare and Social Background of the Tudor and Stuart Banquet*. Ed. C. Anne Wilson. Papers from the First Leeds Symposium on Food History and Traditions, April 1986. Edinburgh. Edinburgh University Press. 60–114.

Brome, Richard. 1640. *The Sparagus Garden: A Comedie*. London. Francis Constable.

Fitzpatrick, Joan. 2007. *Food in Shakespeare: Early Modern Dietaries and the Plays*. Literary and Scientific Cultures of Early Modernity. Aldershot. Ashgate.

Fumerton, Patricia. 1991. *Cultural Aesthetics: Renaissance Literature and the Practice of Social Ornament*. Chicago, IL. University of Chicago Press.

Hamilton, A. C. & others, ed. 1990. *The Spenser Encyclopedia*. Toronto. University of Toronto Press.

Heal, Felicity. 1990. *Hospitality in Early Modern England*. Oxford. Clarendon Press.

Henderson, Paula. 2005. *Tudor House and Garden: Architecture and Landscape in the Sixteenth and Early Seventeenth Centuries*. New Haven, CT, and London. Paul Mellon Centre for Studies in British Art and Yale University Press.

Jeanneret, Michel. 1991. *A Feast of Words: Banquets and Table Talk in the Renaissance*. Trans. Jeremy Whiteley and Emma Hughes. Cambridge. Polity Press.

Lawson, William. 1618. *A New Orchard and Garden ... With the Country Housewifes Garden for Hearbes of Common Vse their Vertues, Seasons, Profits, Ornaments, Varietie of Knots, Models for Trees, and Plots for the Best Ordering of Grounds and Walkes*. London. Nicholas Okes for John Harison.

Markham, Gervase. 1986. *The English Housewife*. Ed. Michael R. Best. Kingston. McGill-Queen's University Press.

Meads, Chris. 2001. *Banquets Set Forth: Banqueting in English Renaissance Drama*. Manchester. Manchester University Press.

Middleton, Thomas & Thomas Dekker. 1999. *The Roaring Girl*. In *Plays on Women*. Ed. Kathleen E. McLuskie and David Bevington. Revels Student Editions. Manchester. Manchester University Press.

National Trust. 2002. *Coughton Court*. Norwich. Jarrold.

Peeters, Clara. 1611. *Still-Life*. Oil on Panel, 52 x 73 cm. Madrid. Museo del Prado.

Richardson, Catherine. 2006. *Domestic Life and Domestic Tragedy in Early Modern England: The Material Life of the Household*. Manchester. Manchester University Press.

Shakespeare, William. 1968. *The First Folio of Shakespeare*. Ed. Charlton Hinman. The Norton Facsimile. New York. Norton.

———. 1982. *The Taming of the Shrew*. Ed. H. J. Oliver. The Oxford Shakespeare. Oxford. Oxford University Press.

————. 2000. *Romeo and Juliet*. Ed. J. L. Levenson. The Oxford Shakespeare. Oxford. Oxford University Press.

Shakespeare, William, and Thomas Middleton. 2004. *Timon of Athens*. Ed. John Jowett. The Oxford Shakespeare. Oxford. Oxford University Press.

————. 2008. *Timon of Athens*. Ed. Anthony B. Dawson and Gretchen E. Minton. London. Arden Shakespeare.

Shepard, Alexandra. 2003. *Meanings of Manhood in Early Modern England*. Oxford. Oxford University Press.

Stead, Jennifer. 1991. 'Bowers of Bliss: The Banquet Setting'. In *'Banquetting Stuffe': The Fare and Social Background of the Tudor and Stuart Banquet*. Ed. C. Anne Wilson. Papers from the First Leeds Symposium on Food History and Traditions, April 1986. Edinburgh. Edinburgh University Press. 115–57.

Steggle, Matthew. 2004. *Richard Brome: Place and Politics on the Caroline Stage*. The Revels Plays Companion Library. Manchester. Manchester University Press.

Van der Hamen, Juan. 1622. *Still-Life of Glass Pottery, and Sweets*. Oil on canvas, 52 x 88 cm. Madrid. Museo del Prado.

Van Dijck, Floris Claesz. 1610. *Still-Life*. Oil on oak panel, 74 x 114 cm (Private Collection).

Wilson, C. Anne. 1991. 'The Evolution of the Banquet Course'. In *'Banquetting Stuffe': The Fare and Social Background of the Tudor and Stuart Banquet*. Ed. C. Anne Wilson. Papers from the First Leeds Symposium on Food History and Traditions, April 1986. Edinburgh. Edinburgh University Press. 9–35.

Chapter 7
'I Must Eat my Dinner':
Shakespeare's Foods from
Apples to Walrus

Joan Fitzpatrick

What do we know about what the early moderns ate and why? Their diet was conditioned by, amongst other factors, rank, location, and humoral theory. Early modern dietaries – prose texts recommending what one should eat and why – can tell us much about attitudes to food and diet in the period. The dietaries are an under-studied resource and yet are important in forming our understanding of what Elizabethans ate, how they regarded specific foods, how consumption differed according to class and nationality, and what audiences might have made of references to food in early modern drama.[1] In the writings of Shakespeare and his contemporaries, a distinct suspicion toward fruit and vegetables is consistent with advice from early modern dietaries that these foods should be consumed with caution. On the other hand, the consumption of animal flesh was broadly encouraged, although certain humoral types were advised to avoid the flesh of specific animals. Via early modern references to specific foods – in the dietaries, in Shakespeare, and in other writings – this essay will focus on the 'dinner' Caliban insists on eating, specifically what his dinner might consist of, and what this might suggest to an early modern audience.

Caliban's assertion about his dinner, taken out of context, suggests a visceral creature who is only interested in satisfying his stomach, but, as critics from Coleridge onwards have noted (Shakespeare 1892, 379–88), he speaks poetically and rationally, and thus presents a more complex figure than merely a compulsion to eat would suggest:

---

[1]   In general, the earliest edition available in English is used as evidence here, although where a subsequent edition adds substantially to the dietary it is preferred. Also, a later edition is preferred over an earlier if it is available as electronic text from the Text Creation Partnership (TCP) at the University of Michigan. Research on the dietaries has been hindered by their frequent use of black-letter typefaces that are hard to read, especially on over-inked leaves with show-through from the previous page. Not only are the electronic texts easier to read but they also enable rapid searches to see how a particular food is represented in each. Some dietaries have indices, but these searches revealed detail easily missed even by the most careful reader, and the Text Creation Partnership is to be applauded for providing scholars with new ways to work on these old books.

CALIBAN I must eat my dinner.
This island's mine, by Sycorax my mother,
Which thou tak'st from me. When thou cam'st first,
Thou strok'st me and made much of me, wouldst give me
Water with berries in 't, and teach me how
To name the bigger light, and how the less,
That burn by day and night; and then I loved thee,
And showed thee all the qualities o' th' isle,
The fresh springs, brine-pits, barren place and fertile –
Cursed be I that did so! All the charms
Of Sycorax, toads, beetles, bats, light on you;
For I am all the subjects that you have,
Which first was mine own king, and here you sty me
In this hard rock, whiles you do keep from me
The rest o' th' island. (1.2.333–46)[2]

But it is this compulsion to eat – a compulsion that does not detract from Caliban's humanity as such, since it is one shared by all humans – that I wish to focus on here. We are not told what Caliban eats for his dinner, but it might well consist of the fruit that grows on the island: the berries he refers to being given by Prospero and which presumably he had found and eaten before Prospero presented them to him in water. Prospero's promise of violence against Caliban also involves food when he tells him: 'Thou shalt be pinched / As thick as honeycomb, each pinch more stinging / Than bees that made 'em' (1.2.330–332), which suggests that Caliban would know what honeycomb is and that he might consume honeycomb and, indeed, the honey produced by the bees on the island. In another promise of violence, this time toward Ferdinand, Prospero tells him:

I'll manacle thy neck and feet together.
Sea-water shalt thou drink; thy food shall be
The fresh-brook mussels, withered roots, and husks
Wherein the acorn cradled. (1.2.464–7)

So, should he wish to consume them, mussels, roots, and acorns are also presumably available to Caliban; but what else might he eat?

In an effort to ingratiate himself with Stephano, Caliban states: 'I'll show thee the best springs; I'll pluck thee berries; / I'll fish for thee, and get thee wood enough' (2.2.159–60) and:

I prithee, let me bring thee where crabs grow,
And I with my long nails will dig thee pig-nuts,
Show thee a jay's nest, and instruct thee how
To snare the nimble marmoset. I'll bring thee
To clust'ring filberts, and sometimes I'll get thee
Young seamews from the rock. Wilt thou go with me? (2.2.166–71)

---

2   All quotations of Shakespeare's plays are from Shakespeare 1989b.

It is not clear whether 'crabs' refers to the crab-apple or the sea creature, and, as Stephen Orgel pointed out, 'it has been invariably assumed' that Shakespeare meant the former 'because of the verb *grow*' where 'crabs would be expected to "dwell"' (Shakespeare 1987, 150n161), but when the term 'crab' is used by Shakespeare, context usually implies that it refers to the fruit. Orgel further notes that 'crabapples were not considered good to eat' because 'their sourness was proverbial' (Shakespeare 1987, 150n161), but this does not mean that they were not eaten or that they would not appeal to Caliban. The 'pig-nuts' referred to by Caliban are the tuber of *Bunium flexuosum*, also termed the 'earth nut' (OED pig-nut 1); and 'filberts' are hazelnuts (OED filbert 1. a.). Reference to the 'jay's nest' might indicate, as Orgel noted, that Caliban is 'offering Stephano the eggs' (Shakespeare 1987, 150n163), but he might be offering to raid the nest for its chicks. Even 'the nimble marmoset' is apparently a reference to food, since the creature was said in Harcourt's *Voyage to Guiana* to be edible (Shakespeare 1961, 68n172). Exactly what it is that Caliban promises to retrieve 'from the rock' has caused much debate, with critics arguing that the word means a kind of bird or fish or limpets (Shakespeare 1892, 138n180). Theobald claimed that Shakespeare could not possibly have meant 'scamell', which appears in the Folio text, and suggested that the correct word was 'shamois', a young kid, or 'sea-malls', a bird that feeds upon fish; he also suggested a bird called a 'stannel', which is a kind of hawk (Shakespeare 1733, 39n19). More recently Benjamin Griffin argued that the word 'scamell' 'is a misreading of 'Seamors', that is *sea-morse* or walrus, which would explain why Caliban specifically offers to get 'young' creatures from the rock; 'Caliban would hardly offer to retrieve a full-grown walrus' (Griffin 2006, 494).

So Caliban's 'dinner' might consist of fruit, specifically berries and perhaps apples, crabs and mussels, honeycomb and honey, nuts, roots, eggs, marmoset, fowl, fish, or even walrus. What would an early modern audience have made of such foods? The following will consider what Shakespeare and his contemporaries, specifically the dietary authors, had to say about these foods, what the early moderns might have considered to be 'missing' from Caliban's dinner, and what they were likely to think he was better off without.

Fruit, vegetables, nuts, and honey

Although wild fruits such as apples, pears, and blackberries had been grown in England for hundreds of years, the early modern period saw the introduction of new fruits – for example apricots, melons, pomegranates – from Southern Europe, which became available for the first time to those who could afford them. So too, dried fruits such as raisins, currants, and figs were imported in large quantities to serve the luxury market. In the writings of Shakespeare and his contemporaries, a distinct suspicion toward fruit in general is consistent with advice from early modern dietaries that fruit should be consumed with caution and in moderation.

In the early modern period it was generally believed that God had ordained animal flesh as fit for human consumption only after the flood (Genesis 9:3). Thomas Moffett notes:

> For whilst Adam and his wife were in Paradise, he had commission to eat only of the fruit of the Garden; being cast thence, he was enjoined to till the ground, and fed in the sweat of his brows upon worts, corn, pulse and roots; but as for flesh, albeit many beasts were slain for sacrifices and apparel, yet none was eaten of men 2240 years after the creation; even till God himself permitted Noah and his family to feed of every sensible thing that moved and lived, as well as of fruits and green herb. (Moffett 1655, E3r–E3v)

Moffett claims that the main reason for man later consuming animal flesh rather than fruit and vegetables alone was a change in man's physical make-up as well as the food typically consumed:

> before the flood men were of stronger constitution, and vegetable fruits grew void of superfluous moisture: so by the flood these were endued with weaker nourishment and men made more subject to violent diseases and infirmities. Whereupon it was requisite or rather necessary, such meat to be appointed for human nourishment, as was in substance and essence most like our own, and might with less loss and labour of natural heat be converted and transubstantiated into our flesh. (E4r)

The notion that fruit was full of water and could cause a harmful imbalance in the body if consumed comes up repeatedly in the dietaries. The dietary author William Vaughan gives a detailed explanation of this view of fruit:

> All fruit for the most part are taken more for wantonness then for any nutritive or necessary good, which they bring unto us. To verifie this, let us but examine with the eye of reason what profit they cause, when they are eaten after meals. Surely we must needs confess, that such eating, which the French call *desert,* is unnaturall, being contrary to physicke or diet: for commonly fruits are of a moist faculty, and therefore fitter to be taken before meals (but corrected with sugar or comfits) than after meales: and then also but very sparingly, least their effects appear to our bodily repentance, which in women grow to be the green sicknesse, in men the morphew, or els some flatuous windy humor. (Vaughan 1612, E4v)

Of course, this did not mean that fruit was not eaten: wild fruit provided free food for the poor, and, as we saw in Tracy Thong's essay in this volume, fruit often appeared as part of a banquet course enjoyed by the better-off, but there was a general consensus that if fruit was to be consumed, not a great deal of it should be eaten and not on a full stomach.

There are numerous references to fruit in Shakespeare, and there tends to be a focus on fruit as inferior or bad. In *The Merchant of Venice*, Antonio welcomes death at the hands of Shylock, comparing himself to 'The weakest kind of fruit' (4.1.114); in *As You Like It*, Touchstone refers to Orlando's verses as 'bad fruit' (3.2. 114); and in *Richard 2*, one of the gardeners complains about the state of the kingdom under Richard's governance:

> our sea-walled garden, the whole land,
> Is full of weeds, her fairest flowers choked up,
> Her fruit trees all unpruned, her hedges ruined ... (3.4.44–6)

In *Hamlet*, Polonius apparently refers to the French fashion of eating fruit after a meal: 'Give first admittance to th' ambassadors. / My news shall be the fruit to that great feast (2.2.51–2). As noted above, Vaughan was dismissive of this French custom, and it seems likely that by comparing Polonius' news – that he has found the cause of Hamlet's lunacy – to fruit, Shakespeare is suggesting that, like the fruit consumed after a meal, this news will do no good.

But what about the apples Caliban might mean when he tells Stephano that he will bring him 'where crabs grow' (2.2.166)? There was some consensus amongst dietary authors that apples should not be eaten raw because they were considered difficult to digest and were thus best eaten either cooked or when ripe or over-ripe.[3] Orgel is correct to assert that 'crabapples were not considered good to eat' because 'their sourness was proverbial' (Shakespeare 1987, 150n161), but this would not have applied to the cooked fruit. The herbalist John Gerard is typical in his view that 'Rosted Apples are alwaies better than the raw, the harm whereof is both mended by the fire, and may also be corrected by adding vnto them seeds or spices' (Gerard & Johnson 1633, Gggggg2v). The dietary author Thomas Cogan also advises against the consumption of raw apples but notes that 'unruly people through wanton appetite will not refrain [from] them, and chiefly in youth when (as it were) by a naturall affection they greedily covet them'. He suggests that apples be eaten 'rosted, or baken, or stewed' and 'with caraways ... or some other kind of comfits' (Cogan 1636, N2v–N3r).

Apples are twice associated with the young or immature in Shakespeare. In *The Tempest*, Gonzalo is made fun of by Sebastian and Antonio when, discussing the recent marriage of the king of Naples' daughter, they quibble over Gonzalo's assertion that Tunis can be equated with Carthage. Antonio asks 'What impossible matter will he make easy next?' to which Sebastian replies 'I think he will carry this island home in his pocket, and give it his son for an apple' (2.1.88–9). It is suggested that Gonzalo does not understand the world around him. It is also possible that Gonzalo is to be imagined exchanging the island for an apple, thus suggesting an ironic inversion: he and not his son is child-like and, specifically, gullible. In *Twelfth Night*, Malvolio describes Cesario as 'Not yet old enough for a man, nor young enough for a boy; as a squash is before 'tis a peascod, or a codling when 'tis almost an apple' (1.5.152–3). The codling is a variety of apple, but 'the name seems to have been applied to a hard kind of apple, not suitable to be eaten raw; hence to any immature or half-grown apple' (OED codling 2. 1.a). Context suggests specific reference to the crab-apple in *The Taming of the Shrew*: it is presumably what Katherine has in mind when she refers to the sourness of the crab (2.1.226–8). It is also what is meant by Robin Goodfellow when, in *A Midsummer Night's Dream*, he reports on the tricks he likes to play upon others:

---

[3]   The 'apple-john', a distinct variety of apple, was said to keep for two years and be in perfection when shriveled and withered (OED apple-john).

And sometime lurk I in a gossip's bowl
In very likeness of a roasted crab,
And when she drinks, against her lips I bob,
And on her withered dewlap pour the ale. (2.1.47–50)

The 'crab' referred to is probably the crab-apple, because an apple would be more likely than a crab to 'bob' in water.

An audience might be expected to associate apples with childishness, impetuous youth, and unruly, wanton appetite, characteristics that are especially pertinent to Caliban, who is naive enough to believe that Stephano would make a good master and whose wanton appetite is evident in his attempted rape of Miranda and possibly also in his eagerness to drink the wine offered to him by Stephano. If Caliban is to be imagined eating raw apples, then it might well be suggested that he is harming himself through this ill-advised diet; such a diet would, by extension, also harm others, since it was believed (rightly, as it turned out) that what one ate affected behaviour. Of course, it is possible that Caliban would realize that apples should be cooked, since he has already benefited from the influence of culture in Prospero's preparation of the raw materials that exist on the island: the berries that are put into water to form a kind of fruit-juice.

The generic term 'berries', as well as references to specific types of the fruit, occurs several times in Shakespeare. As Vaughan and Vaughan indicated, the drink Prospero gives Caliban might allude to that made from cedar-berries and drunk by those who survived the shipwreck in Strachey's account of Bermuda – an account which likely influenced Shakespeare when writing *The Tempest* – or perhaps it is wine, since 'grapes' was 'a synonym for berries, especially in Old English' (Shakespeare 1999, 173–4n335). Significantly, although Prospero presented Caliban with 'Water with berries in't' (1.2.334), Caliban offers to 'pluck ... berries' for Stephano, with no suggestion that they will be prepared in the same manner; it is not clear whether Caliban is unable or unwilling to prepare the berries as he has been shown, but Prospero later says that he is 'a born devil, on whose nature / Nurture can never stick' (4.1.188–9). Elsewhere in Shakespeare, eating berries suggests a kind of animalistic feeding or at least a feeding that is unsophisticated and especially close to the natural world, although this is problematised by context. In *Timon of Athens*, the First Thief complains to Timon: 'We cannot live on grass, on berries, water, / As beasts and birds and fishes', but Timon's reply suggests that the thieves are more barbaric than they realize and that it is not their diet of berries that defines them but their attitude to humanity: 'Nor on the beasts themselves, the birds and fishes; / You must eat men' (4.3.424–7). In *Titus Andronicus*, Aaron tells the child created by himself and Tamora:

Come on, you thick-lipped slave, I'll bear you hence,
For it is you that puts us to our shifts.
I'll make you feed on berries and on roots,
And fat on curds and whey, and suck the goat,
And cabin in a cave, and bring you up
To be a warrior and command a camp. (4.2.174–9)

The animalistic nature of the child's diet, reinforced by the use of the words 'feed', 'fat', and 'suck', are undercut by the fact that he will be nurtured as a commander of men.

Aaron's bastard child will feed 'on roots', a foodstuff also available to Caliban on the island, since Prospero tells Ferdinand that he will be compelled to eat 'withered roots' (1.2.466). In *Timon of Athens*, Timon's foraging for roots would have struck an early modern audience as distinctly bestial, indeed pig-like. Ruth Morse observed that here 'Timon's world has narrowed to the point where only food counts, and that food the lowest and least appropriate food fit for men, roots' (Morse 1983, 146). Presumably, Prospero would think such a foodstuff fit for Caliban, whom he regards as animalistic, describing him as 'A freckled whelp, hag-born – not honoured with / A human shape' (1.2. 284–5); indeed there is a suggestion that Prospero regards Caliban as distinctly pig-like, since Caliban complains 'here you sty me / In this hard rock' (1.2.344–5), the term 'sty' usually used in reference to pigs (OED sty *v*. 2). Yet as with the berries – food in its raw state that is prepared by Prospero – roots do not of themselves suggest bestiality and might benefit from the application of culture. This happens in *Cymbeline*, when Innogen, disguised as Fidele, prepares food for her brothers and Belarius in a cave in rural Wales:

> GUIDERIUS But his neat cookery!
> [BELARIUS] He cut our roots in characters,
> And sauced our broths as Juno had been sick
> And he her dieter. (4.2.50–53)

To present the roots as letters of the alphabet does more than Roger Warren suggests in his comparison with modern alphabet soup. The characters not only 'make the food more interesting [for children] and so tempt them to eat' (Shakespeare 1998, 196n51) but blur the distinction between nature and culture in much the same way that Caliban's assertion that he must eat his dinner, suggesting the visceral, is undercut by the articulate and reasoned outburst that immediately follows. Eating roots also suggests simplicity. Before Timon's friends abandon him, the misanthropic Apemantus warns Timon to beware of culinary indulgence:

> Here's that which is too weak to be a sinner:
> Honest water, which ne'er left man i' th' mire.
> This and my food are equals; there's no odds.
> Feasts are too proud to give thanks to the gods. (1.2. 57–60)

For Apemantus, the eating of basic food signals a healthy distance from the corruption located in sophisticated feasts that require money and preparation as opposed to food in its natural state, something that Timon shows he has learned when he presents his parody of a feast: the meal of stones and steaming water that he places before his false friends. As John Jowett pointed out, 'stones and water can be seen as equivalent to the bread and wine of the Communion. Christ's first miracle was to turn water to wine, and in the desert Satan tempted Christ to "command this stone that it be made bread" (John 2:1–11; Luke 4:3)' (Shakespeare & Middleton 2004, 257n84.2). When Apemantus states 'Rich men sin, and I eat root' (1.2. 70), we get the message that sinners eat fancy foods, specifically food that has been prepared. If we apply this logic to *The Tempest*, then Caliban's offer to gather berries for Stephano is not inferior to the preparation of berries in water presented to Caliban by Prospero; indeed, Shakespeare is suggesting quite the opposite.

Caliban also offers to dig nuts for Stephano, and Prospero says he will force Ferdinand to eat the husks of the acorn. Nuts are mentioned numerous times in Shakespeare, but of the specific nuts available on the island, it is only the acorn that appears elsewhere in the plays as a foodstuff. In Shakespeare's time, acorns were generally considered fit only for animal-feed, although it seems that humans still ate acorns when food was scarce. It was thought that acorns were ordinarily eaten by humans in the Golden Age but were replaced by cereal crops and, thus, bread. Acorns were usually fed to pigs, but other animals also benefited: the dietary author William Vaughan advises 'You may feed turkeys with bruised acorns, and they will prosper exceedingly' (Vaughan 1612, D4v). Francis Bacon was typical in the view that 'Acornes were good till bread was found' (Bacon 1639, Aa7v), a point also made by the dietary author Levinus Lemnius:

> Men well enough know the Beech ... and other mast trees, which in the old time (before the invention of tillage and the use of corne) ministred competent food and nourishment. Whereupon afterward grew a proverb; It is a mere folly, when we have corn, still to eat acorns. (Lemnius 1587, P5v)

Roger Ascham believed that for men to eat acorns was barbaric: 'But now, when men know the difference, and have the examples, both of the best, and of the worst, surely, to follow rather the *Goths* in Ryming, than the Greekes in true versifiyng, were even to eate acorns with swine, when we may freely eate wheat bread amongst men' (Ascham 1570, R4r). In Thomas Heywood's play *The Golden Age*, the Clown claims that Saturn – the new king who has usurped his elder brother Tytan upon the death of their father Uranus – has many virtues: 'he hath taught his people to sow, to plow, to reape corne, and to skorne Akehornes with their heeles, to bake and to brue [brew]: we that were wont to drinke nothing but water, haue the brauest liquor at Court as passeth' (Heywood 1611, B4r). However, Holinshed points out that the poor often had little choice about what to eat:

> The bread through out the land is made of such graine as the soile yeeldeth, neverthelesse the gentilitie commonlie provide themselues sufficientlie of wheat for their owne tables, whilest their household and poor neighbours in some shires are inforced to content themselues with rie, or barlie, yea and in time of dearth manie with bread made either of beans, peason, or otes, or of altogither and some acornes among, of which scourge the poorest doo soonest tast, sith they are least able to prouide themselues of better. (Holinshed 1587, P5v)

Thomas Cogan compares acorns to chestnuts and notes that Galen was ambivalent about them but that if roasted they 'will soone stay a laske [looseness of the bowels], as I learned of an old woman, which therewith did great cures in the flix [flux]' (Cogan 1636, Q1r).

Acorns seem to have been ordinarily eaten by humans in early modern Spain: the herbalist John Gerard cites Carolus Clusius or Charles de L'Écluse, the influential sixteenth-century horticulturist, who reported that 'the Acorne is esteemed of, eaten, and brought into the market to be sold, in the city of Salamanca in Spaine, and in many other places of that countrey ... Moreouer, at this day in Spain the Acorne is serued for a second course' (Gerard & Johnson 1633, Vuuuu5r). But in England, only the poor ate acorns and only when necessity compelled them.

In *As You Like It*, the love-sick Orlando, spread out under a tree and described by Celia as 'like a dropped acorn' (3.2.227), is, according to Rosalind, fruit dropped from 'Jove's tree' (3.2.231). The allusion is to the Golden Age when men 'Did live by ... apples, nuts and pears ... And by the acorns dropped on ground, from Jove's broad tree' (Ovid 1916, 1, 119–21) but also to the New Testament: 'A good tree cannot bring forth evil fruit, neither can a corrupt tree bring forth good fruit' (Matthew 7:18). The Forest of Ardenne is a kind of Golden World, but it is one informed by the Christian ideals of charity and forgiveness.

The low status afforded to acorns in early modern culture would explain why Prospero forcing Ferdinand to eat the mere husks of the acorn is so severe a test of his love for Miranda. Caliban has access to acorns, and eating them would further reinforce his bestiality, as does offering to dig nuts from the ground for Stephano. The connection between eating acorns and bestial impulses is evident in *Cymbeline* when Posthumus imagines that the chaste Innogen has had sex with his Italian rival:

> This yellow Giacomo in an hour – was 't not? –
> Or less – at first? Perchance he spoke not, but
> Like a full-acorned boar, a German one,
> Cried 'O!' and mounted; found no opposition
> But what he looked for should oppose and she
> Should from encounter guard. (2.5.14–19)

As Roger Warren pointed out, 'In Topsell's *History of Four-footed Beasts* (1607), the swine of Lower Germany are said to be "fierce, strong, and very fat" (p. 514). The phrase suggests the gross animalism of Giacomo's intercourse with Innogen' (Shakespeare 1998, 151n168). That Giacomo is Italian is perhaps also relevant: as Gerard noted above, the Catholic Spanish ate acorns, and Shakespeare's audience might be expected to have spotted connections being made here between mere animals and the Italians who, like the Spanish, are religious and political rivals. Female sexual continence also preoccupies Prospero in *The Tempest*: in his desire to test Ferdinand in case 'too light winning' of his daughter' might 'make the prize light' (1.2.454–5); and his disgust at Caliban's attempted rape of her, an attempt he gleefully admits: 'O ho, O ho! Would 't had been done! / Thou didst prevent me; I had peopled else / This isle with Calibans (1.2.351–3).

Caliban does not mention honey, but Prospero does when he tells him: 'Thou shalt be pinched / As thick as honeycomb, each pinch more stinging / Than bees that made 'em' (1.2.330–332), so honeycomb and honey is a likely source of food on the island. Honeycomb does not appear elsewhere in Shakespeare, and in the dietaries it is honey rather than honeycomb that features. Honey is generally praised for its medicinal powers and for being nutritious. Thomas Elyot's is typical of the views expressed about the food: 'Honey as well in meat as in drink, is of incomparable efficacy: for it not only cleanseth, altereth, and nourisheth, but also it long time preserveth that uncorrupted, which is put into it ...', and he continues, 'Of this excellent matter, most wonderfully wrought and gathered by a little bee, as well of the pure dew of heaven as of the most subtile humour of sweet and vertuous herbs & flowers, bee made liquors commodious to mankind, as mead, metheglin, and oximel' (Elyot 1595, H4r–H4v). Yet, as with most foods, it seems that the humor of the person consuming the honey ought to be taken into account, at least according to William Bullein, who noted, 'honey is hot and dry in the second degree, and does cleanse very much, and is a medicinable mea[t] most chiefliest for old men and women. For it doth warm them & convert the[m] into good blood' but he warns that it 'It is not good for cholerick persons because of the heat and dryness' (Bullein 1558, P7v).

Shakespeare too was ambivalent about honey. As Gordon Williams noted, honey was a synonym for 'sexual sweets' and could also refer to semen and the vagina (Williams 1994, 'honey'). Shakespeare repeatedly refers to honey's sweetness, but often in the context of sexual indulgence. For example, in *Troilus and Cressida*, Priam tells Paris that while he is distracted by Helen, others must fight: 'Like one besotted on your sweet delights. / You have the honey still, but these the gall' (2.2.142–3); in *Titus Andronicus*, Tamora tells her boys, Chiron and Demetrius, to get rid of Lavinia after they have enjoyed her sexually: 'But when ye have the honey ye desire / Let not this wasp outlive, us both to sting' (2.3.131–2); and in *The Rape of Lucrece*, Tarquin, before his attack upon Lucrece, tells her 'I know what thorns the growing rose defends; / I think the honey guarded with a sting' (492–3), and afterwards she laments on behalf of her husband Collatine: 'In thy weak hive a wandering wasp hath crept, / And sucked the honey which thy chaste bee kept' (839–40). Ironically, it is Caliban's failure to rape Miranda that results in pinches 'As thick as honeycomb' and 'more stinging / Than bees that made 'em' (1.2.331–2); here honey and bees suggest not sex but the consequences of seeking it.

Flesh, Fish, and Fowl

What might an early modern audience have made of the suggestion that Caliban eats the marmoset or monkeys that populate the island? Those playgoers who knew what a marmoset was would have found the notion of eating monkey-flesh exotic, and it is unlikely they would have had any experience of it; the same is true of 'seamors', that is, seamorse or walrus (if Benjamin Griffin is correct and that is what is meant by 'scamels'), but they ate the flesh of other animals with enthusiasm when they could afford it. In the early modern period, the consumption of animal flesh was encouraged: the standard early modern view, as discussed above, appears to have been that eating meat was divinely ordained and more healthy than a vegetarian diet, although there were lots of factors to be taken into consideration before consuming it, including whether or not a specific meat was suited to one's humour, occupation, and even nationality.[4] As Erica Fudge noted, the eating of animal flesh 'held a more powerful position in theological terms than any attempt to regain the vegetarian innocence of Eden', since such a diet signified human dominion over animals. A vegetarian diet 'would take away a point of humiliation for humans that was vital to their understanding of their place in the universe', where the eating of animal flesh 'represents both death (human mortality) and power (human dominion)' (Fudge 2004, 75). However, the eating of monkey-flesh might have struck an early modern audience as unnerving, given the disconcerting physical similarities between man and ape. As James Knowles pointed out, 'the ape raised questions about the boundaries of the human and animal, a highly uncertain and contested limen. There existed a real fear that men (and, more likely, women and boys) might easily continue the postlapsarian trajectory of decay and metamorphose toward the animal' (Knowles 2004, 139). Anthony Pagden noted that Europeans who travelled to the New World were disturbed by native eating habits: 'the Indians not only ate men, who were too high in the scale of being to be food, they also ate creatures which were too low', something that 'was a sure sign of their barbarism because by such unselective consumption the Indian revealed ... his inability to recognise the division between species in the natural world and the proper purpose of each one' (Pagden 1982, 87; Fudge 2004, 79).

Aside from the marmoset, no mention is made of eating animal flesh in *The Tempest*, but Caliban tells Stephano 'I'll fish for thee' (2.2.160). Fish was generally considered inferior to animal flesh, specifically red meat, because it was believed to be less nourishing. 'Fish days', implemented for economic reasons – to encourage the fishing industry and bring down the high price of meat – were apparently unpopular. For many Protestants, eating fish was associated with Catholicism, specifically the practice of abstaining from animal flesh on Fridays. The fish was an early Christian symbol, and the connection between fish-eating and Christ, especially via the biblical story of Christ's miraculous multiplying of loaves and fishes (Mark 6:35–42), was used by some Catholics to suggest that eating fish was superior to eating animal flesh. As Edward Jeninges indicates in his prose tract promoting the eating of fish and the fishing industry, many people considered laws

---

[4]   Beef is an interesting example: Andrew Boorde claims that 'Beefe is good meate for an Englyssh man' if it is of a high quality and if it comes from a young, male cow. He asserts that old beef and the flesh of cows causes melancholy and leprosy, but if the meat is well salted, in order to get rid of thick blood, 'it doth make an Englysshe man stro[n]ge the educacyon of him with it co[n]sydered' (Boorde 1547, F1v–F2r). William Bullein also thought that beef should be young and male and that it is difficult to digest. He specifies that the meat that should be consumed by those engaged in manual labour and that 'Much béefe customably eaten of idle persons, and nice folkes that labour not, bringeth many diseases ...' (Bullein 1595, I4v).

advocating abstinence from the eating of meat reminiscent of those 'made and used in the time of Papistrie, and by ancient authoritie of the Pope, who we should not in anything imitate, but rather in all thinges by contrarie' (Jeninges 1590, D3r); it does not follow, argues Jeninges, that this law is wrong, since 'many good lawes and ordinances in the time of Papistrie was by them made and ordained' (D3v). Discussing the relative merits of flesh and fish, Thomas Moffett criticizes those 'filthy Friars' who think fish superior to meat because Christ fed upon it, arguing that Christ himself adhered to the laws of Moses and forbade the Israelites to eat fish with neither scales nor fins (Moffett 1655, H3r). In the monasteries, meat was only eaten occasionally: the Benedictine Rule stated 'let the use of fleshmeat be granted to the sick who are very weak, for the restoration of their strength; but, as soon as they are better, let all abstain from fleshmeat as usual' (Benedict 1952, 91; chapter 36). Thomas Moffett concludes that 'all fish (compared with flesh) is cold and moist, of little nourishment, engendring watrish and thinn blood' (Moffett 1655, U1v); and William Bullein, citing Galen, claims 'the nourishments of flesh is better than the nourishments of fish' (Bullein 1595, K5v).

Fish is referred to repeatedly in Shakespeare. In *2 Henry 4*, Sir John criticizes Prince John for eating 'many fish meals' (4.2.89), thus suggesting that he is weak. Denouncing Prince John for eating fish would be in keeping with the historical figure upon whom Sir John was apparently based: the proto-Protestant martyr Oldcastle. In *King Lear*, the disguised Kent says to Lear

> I do profess to be no less than I seem, to serve him truly that will put me in trust, to love him that is honest, to converse with him that is wise and says little, to fear judgement, to fight when I cannot choose, and to eat no fish. (1.4.13–17)

As Stanley Wells pointed out, the reference to eating no fish is 'Self-deflatingly anticlimactic' but might also suggest that Kent is 'a loyal Protestant who does not fast on Fridays' (Shakespeare 2000, 126n14–15) or, as Gordon Williams noted, that he avoids the company of whores; fish was often associated with sex, specifically female flesh and genitalia (Williams 1994, 'fish'). In *Hamlet*, the prince calls Polonius 'a fishmonger' (2.2.170) before asking him 'have you a daughter?' (2.2.179). Critics often interpret this as Hamlet calling Polonius a bawd or a pander, but Harold Jenkins argued convincingly that it demonstrates Hamlet's antipathy to mating and procreation due to 'the supposition that the womenfolk of fishmongers have a special aptitude for procreation' (Jenkins 1975, 117). In John Marston's *The Dutch Courtesan*, Mary Faugh announces that although she is a member of the Family of Love, a sinner, and considered a bawd she is 'none of the wicked that eat fish o' Fridays' (Marston 1997, 1.2.19–20), which suggests that for all her faults at least she is not Catholic.

Although Caliban might be referring to fruit when he tells Stephano 'I prithee, let me bring thee where crabs grow' (2.2.166), he might be referring to the sea-creature, and Prospero mentions 'The fresh-brook mussels' (1.2. 466) Ferdinand will eat and which would also be available to Caliban. According to William Bullein, 'Crauises [crayfishes] and crabs be very good fishes, the meat of them doth help the lungs, but they be hurtful for the bladder, yet they will engender seed'.

With 'seed', that is semen (OED seed *n.* 4), there is the same association with sex that we have seen for fish. Bullein warns that 'muscles and oysters would be well boiled, roasted, or baked with onions, wine, butter, sugar, ginger, and pepper, or else they be very windy and phlegmatic. Choleric stomachs may well digest raw oysters, but they have cast many a one away' (Bullein 1558, P4r). Thomas Cogan thought crab, lobster, and shrimp 'of the same nature' as crayfish, which he thought very nourishing, and 'doth not lightly corrupt in the stomacke. Yet is it hard of digestion ...' (Cogan 1636, Y1v).

Crab is referred to by Shakespeare in the plays but not explicitly as a foodstuff. In *Love's Labour's Lost* and *Hamlet*, the focus is on the action of the crab: Hamlet refers to the crab going backward (2.2.205–6) and Holofernes to the crab falling (4.2.3–7). Crab is also the name of Launce's dog in *The Two Gentlemen of Verona*, which might be a comment upon his character: he is crabbed, that is, froward. The only other reference to mussels occurs in *The Merry Wives of Windsor*, where Falstaff calls Simple 'mussel-shell', which T. W. Craik explained as follows: 'Either because Simple is gaping in expectation', as noted by Samuel Johnston in his 1765 edition of the plays, 'or because he is insignificant', as noted by H. C. Hart in his 1904 Arden edition of the play (Shakespeare 1989a, 197n26).

The notion that crabs will encourage the generation of sperm is pertinent to Caliban, as is the belief that mussels must be well cooked. Again there is an association between the food Caliban eats and his sexual potency, something that is a direct threat to Miranda, and again the issue of whether of not Caliban prepares his food or eats it in a raw state is pertinent.

Birds and Eggs

It is not clear whether Caliban eats birds, the young of birds, or their eggs. As Stephen Orgel noted, Caliban's reference to the 'jay's nest' might indicate the bird's eggs (Shakespeare 1987, 150n163), but he might also be alluding to its young, whilst the 'seamew' is a seagull but other meanings are possible. As mentioned earlier, Theobald suggested that 'scamel' is a printer's error for 'shamois', meaning a young kid, specifically an antelope, or 'sea-mews', a bird that feeds upon fish, or that it might mean 'stannel', a kind of hawk. Theobald further noted, 'It is no matter which of the three readings we embrace, so we take a word signifying something in nature' (Shakespeare 1733, 39n19). But it might well matter which kind of bird was intended.

The dietary authors were not full of praise for wild birds. Thomas Cogan was of the opinion that 'tame birds (as Isaack saith) do nourish more than the wylde, and be more temperate' (Cogan 1636, T3r). William Bullein on the subject of 'the flesh of herons, bittors, and shouellers' announced:

> These fowles bee fishers, and be very rawe, and fleugmaticke, like vnto the meate whereof they are fedde: the young be best, and ought to bee eaten with pepper, synnamom [cinnamon], sugar and ginger, and drinke wine after them for good digestion: and thus do for al water foules. (Bullein 1595, K3r–3v)

If, as Theobald suggested, 'scamel' is a printer's error for 'stannel', a kind of hawk, then a colonial dimension is added to Caliban's choice of foodstuff. Fynes Moryson, discussing the effects of Lord Deputy Mountjoy's campaign against Irish rebels in 1602, describes how burning the rebels' corn reduced them to cannibalism and forced them to eat other undesirable foods '... they besides fed not onely on Hawkes, Kytes, and vnsavourie birds of prey, but on Horseflesh, and other things vnfit for mans feeding' (Moryson 1617, Bbb2r). There is a sense in which the extenuating circumstances of the famine become obscured by the fulfilment of what the English suspected all along, that the Irish are savages; later in his description of the Irish diet Moryson is appalled that they seem to enjoy the taste of horse-flesh (Moryson 1617, Sss2v). If Caliban is to be imagined consuming what Bullein termed 'water fowl', then an early modern audience would presumably have thought him less savage than if, like the Irish, he eats hawkes. The only gulls that appear in Shakespeare are human fools, and, not surprisingly, there is no reference to eating hawk.[5]

When Shakespeare refers to 'fowl' as a foodstuff, the term is often used in the context of hunting, and there is usually a distinct sympathy for the bird. In *Measure For Measure*, Isabella's response to the news that her brother Claudio will die 'tomorrow' is 'O, that's sudden! Spare him, spare him! / He's not prepared for death. Even for our kitchens / We kill the fowl of season' (2.2.85–7). She later refers to Angelo as one who 'Nips youth i' th' head and follies doth enew / As falcon doth the fowl' (3.1. 89–90). In *Much Ado About Nothing*, Benedick says of the lovesick Claudio, 'Alas, poor hurt fowl, now will he creep into sedges' (2.1. 190–191), and later Benedick is the fowl 'stalked' by Claudio and his friends when they discuss within his hearing how Beatrice is in love with him (2.3.93). Sir John Falstaff describes the men he has recruited for battle in *1 Henry 4* to be 'as such as fear the report of a caliver [gun] worse than a struck fowl or a hurt wild duck' (4.2.19–21). The innocent Lucrece, when confronted in her bed by the rapist Tarquin, is compared to the fowl that trembles for fear of the falcon (*The Rape of Lucrece* 505–12).

If Caliban intends to steal the jay's young from their nest, then this would suggest an unnatural barbarity, a behaviour that is clearly uncultured; certainly both the chicks and the eggs would have been considered strange foods in the period, and, as is clear from references to 'fowl', it seems that Shakespeare was alert to the cruelty of any living creature being hunted and killed. As I have argued elsewhere (Fitzpatrick 2007, 57–67; 76–80), Shakespeare may have had what his contemporaries would have considered a strange sympathy for vegetarianism, especially in those plays where pastoralism features. In *As You Like it*, Duke Senior and his followers hunt animals for food, but the shepherds who also live in the forest do not. Corin's focus is on the self-contained industry of the pastoral life and the pleasure he gains from witnessing the nourishment of his flock: 'Sir, I am a true labourer. I earn that I eat, get that I wear; owe no man hate, envy no man's happiness; glad of other men's good, content with my harm; and the greatest of my

---

[5]   For example, Malvolio is referred to as a gull in *Twelfth Night* (3.2.65); a 'gull' was also a joke or trick, as in *Much Ado About Nothing* (2.3.117).

pride is to see my ewes graze and my lambs suck' (3.2.71–5). Corin does not kill his sheep for food but, rather, facilitates their feeding. It is only those courtiers who misunderstand the essence of pastoral life who eat meat. So too in *The Winter's Tale*, those most in tune with pastoral living do not consume the flesh of animals: when the Clown is sent by Perdita to get ingredients for the sheep-shearing feast, his shopping list suggests that the feast will be vegetarian (4.3.35–48).

So what does Caliban's diet tell us about Shakespeare's conception of him and what an early modern audience might have made of this curious figure? Berries and roots, at first glance, suggest the bestial, but upon closer examination these foods are amenable to culture via preparation. The same is true of apples, which are associated with wanton youth, especially when raw, but are less harmful if cooked. So too Caliban problematises simplistic notions of barbarism versus culture, as is evident when demands about filling his stomach are quickly followed with an eloquent and reasoned outburst against Prospero's violence. Shakespeare's sympathy for hunted animals would suggest that killing the marmoset, the walrus, or wild fowl for food is barbaric, but consuming fish was also problematic since it was considered less healthy than animal flesh and was also considered a 'Catholic' food. Caliban's consumption of fish and perhaps also acorns might, for a typical early modern playgoer, align him with the religious and political enemy, as would the hawk that Theobald suggested is meant by 'stannel'. Crab-meat and honey were considered healthy: eating crab was thought to enhance sexual potency, but that is worrying in a would-be rapist, and honey too was aligned with sex and sexual fluids. A recurrent feature here is ambivalence toward the foods represented in the play which in turn signals ambivalence toward Caliban himself: in the final analysis, Caliban is neither clearly bestial nor clearly cultured.

Works Cited

Ascham, Roger. 1570. *The Scholemaster or Plaine and Perfite Way of Teachyng Children, to Vnderstand, Write, and Speake, the Latin Tong*. STC 832. London. John Daye.

Bacon, Francis. 1639. *The Essayes Or, Counsels, Ciuill and Morall ... With a Table of the Colours, or Apparances of Good and Euill*. STC 1151. London. John Beale.

Benedict, Saint. 1952. *The Rule of Saint Benedict: In Latin and English*. Trans. and ed. Justin McCann. Orchard Books. London. Burns Oates.

Boorde, Andrew. 1547. *Compendious Regiment or a Dietary of Health*. STC 3380. London. Wyllyam Powell.

Bullein, William. 1558. *A New Book Entitled the Government of Health*. STC 4039. London. John Day.

———. 1595. *The Gouernment of Health: a Treatise ... for the Especiall Good and Healthfull Preseruation of Mans Bodie from All Noysome Diseases, Proceeding By the Excesse of Euill Diet, and Other Infirmities of Nature: Full of Excellent Medicines, and Wise Counsels, for Conseruation of Health, in Men, Women, and Children*. STC 4042. London. Valentine Sims.

Cogan, Thomas. 1636. *The Haven of Health*. STC 5484. London. Anne Griffin for Roger Ball.

Elyot, Thomas. 1595. *The Castell of Health, Corrected, and in Some Places Augmented By the First Author Thereof*. STC 7656. London. The Widdow Orwin for Matthew Lownes.

Fitzpatrick, Joan. 2007. *Food in Shakespeare: Early Modern Dietaries and the Plays*. Literary and Scientific Cultures of Early Modernity. Aldershot. Ashgate.

Fudge, Erica. 2004. 'Saying Nothing Concerning the Same: On Dominion, Purity, and Meat in Early Modern England'. Trans. Edward Babcock. In *Renaissance Beasts: Of Animals, Humans, and Other Wonderful Creatures*. Edited by Erica Fudge. Urbana. University of Illinois Press. 70–86.

Gerard, John, and Thomas Johnson. 1633. *The Herball or Generall Historie of Plantes. Gathered By Iohn Gerarde of London Master in Chirurgerie Very Much Enlarged and Amended By Thomas Iohnson Citizen and Apothecarye of London*. STC 11751. London. Adam Islip, Joyce Norton, and Richard Whitakers.

Griffin, Benjamin. 2006. 'Emending Caliban's "Scamels"'. *Notes and Queries*. 251. 494–5.

Heywood, Thomas. 1611. *The Golden Age. Or The Liues of Jupiter and Saturne, with the Deifying of the Heathen Gods*. STC 13325. London. [Nicholas Okes] for William Barrenger.

Holinshed, Raphael. 1587. *Chronicles, Newlie Augmented and Continued By J. Hooker Alias Vowell Gent. and Others*. STC 13569. Vol. 1: *The Description of Britaine; The Description of England; The Historie of England*. 3 vols. London. [H. Denham,] at the expenses of J. Harison, G. Bishop, R. Newberie, H. Denham, and T. Woodcocke.

Jeninges, Edward. 1590. *A Briefe Discouery of the Damages That Happen to This Realme By Disordered and Vnlawfull Diet. The Benefites and Commodities That Otherwaies Might Ensue. With a Perswasion of the People: for a Better Maintenance to the Nauie*. STC 14486. London. Roger Ward.

Jenkins, Harold. 1975. 'Hamlet and the Fishmonger'. In *Deutsche Shakespeare-Gesellschaft West Jahrbuch*. Edited by Hermann Heuer, Ernst Theodor Sehrt, and Rudolf Stamm. Heidelberg. Quelle and Meyer. 109–20.

Knowles, James. 2004. '"Can ye Not Tell a Man from a Marmoset?" Apes and Others on the Early Modern Stage'. In *Renaissance Beasts: Of Animals, Humans, and Other Wonderful Creatures*. Edited by Erica Fudge. Urbana. University of Illinois Press. 138–63.

Lemnius, Levinus. 1587. *An Herbal for the Bible*. Trans. Thomas Newton. STC 15454. London. Edmund Bollifant.

Marston, John. 1997. *The Dutch Courtesan*. Ed. David Crane. The New Mermaids. London. A&C Black.

Moffett, Thomas. 1655. *Healths Improvement: Or, Rules Comprizing and Discovering the Nature, Method, and Manner of Preparing All Sorts of Food Used in This Nation*. 1st ed. Wing M2382. London. Tho[mas]: Newcomb for Samuel Thomson.

Morse, Ruth. 1983. 'Unfit for Human Consumption: Shakespeare's Unnatural Food'. In *Jahrbuch der Deutschen Shakespeare-Gesellschaft West*. 125–49.

Moryson, Fynes. 1617. *An Itinerary Written By Fynes Moryson Gent. (Containing His Ten Yeeres Travell Through the Twelve Dominions of Germany, Bohmerland, ... France, England, Scotland, and Ireland)*. STC 18205. London. J. Beale.

Ovid. 1916. *Metamorphoses*. Trans. Frank Justus Miller. Vol. 2. 2 vols. London. William Heinemann.

Pagden, Anthony. 1982. *The Fall of Natural Man: The American Indian and the Origins of Comparative Ethnology*. Cambridge. Cambridge University Press.

Shakespeare, William, and Thomas Middleton. 2004. *Timon of Athens*. Ed. John Jowett. The Oxford Shakespeare. Oxford. Oxford University Press.

———. 1733. *The Works of Shakespeare*. Ed. Lewis Theobald. London. A. Bettesworth and C. Hitch [and] J. Tonson [etc.].

———. 1892. *A New Variorum Edition of Shakespeare*. Ed. Horace Howard Furness. Vol. 9: *The Tempest*. 27 vols. London. J. B. Lippincott.

———. 1961. *The Tempest*. Ed. Frank Kermode. The Arden Shakespeare. London. Methuen.

———. 1987. *The Tempest*. Ed. Stephen Orgel. The Oxford Shakespeare. Oxford. Oxford University Press.

———. 1989a. *The Merry Wives of Windsor*. Ed. T. W. Craik. Oxford. Oxford University Press.

———. 1989b. *The Complete Works*. Ed. Stanley Wells, Gary Taylor, John Jowett, William Montgomery. Prepared by William Montgomery and Lou Burnard. Oxford. Oxford Electronic Publishing, Oxford University Press.

———. 1998. *Cymbeline*. Ed. Roger Warren. The Oxford Shakespeare. Oxford. Oxford University Press.

———. 1999. *The Tempest*. Ed. Virginia Mason Vaughan and Alden T. Vaughan. The Arden Shakespeare: Third Series. London. Arden Shakespeare.

———. 2000. *The History of King Lear*. Ed. Stanley Wells. The Oxford Shakespeare. Oxford. Oxford University Press.

Vaughan, William. 1612. *Natural and Artificial Directions for Health, Derived from the Best Philosophers, as Well Modern, as Ancient ... Newly Corrected and Augmented By the Author*. STC 24615. London. T. S[nodham] for Roger Jackson.

Williams, Gordon. 1994. *A Dictionary of Sexual Language and Imagery in Shakespearean and Stuart Literature*. Vol. 1: A–F. 3 vols. London. Athlone.

———. 1994. *A Dictionary of Sexual Language and Imagery in Shakespearean and Stuart Literature*. Vol. 2: G–P. 3 vols. London. Athlone.

Chapter 8
Narrative and Dramatic Sauces: Reflections upon Creativity, Cookery, and Culinary Metaphor in Some Early Seventeenth-Century Dramatic Prologues

Chris Meads

Thomas Carew, for William Davenant, in 1634, addressed 'The Reader' of *The Wits*, claiming that theatre can be metaphorically allied with cookery and entertainment of a culinary nature:

> It hath been said of old, that plays are feasts,
> Poets the cooks, and the spectators guests. (Davenant 1968, vol. 2 165)

Whether Carew alludes to a lost proverb has proved impossible to ascertain; he seems more likely to have been acknowledging a theatrically generated adage which achieved a proverbial dimension through its currency over time. The shared qualities of the poet and the cook in terms of their capacity for creative metamorphosis and the particular discipline of cooking alongside that of writing proved irresistible to the writers of these prologues to be dealt with below. Michel Jeanneret's analysis, particularly in relation to the prose of Rabelais, and to Montaigne in *A Feast of Words: Des mets et des mots. Banquets et propos de table a la Renaissance*, rendered one alive to the way in which table talk, talk about food, and the literary representation of feasting married the word to food in a fundamental and irrevocable fashion for Renaissance thinkers. The mouth that eats is the mouth that talks, and also that which speaks the lines created by the writer. It is the mouth that tastes, too, and the use of the metaphor of taste, as in both delight for the palate and the critical judgement of an audience, also occurs in these prologues and addresses to auditors from the early seventeenth century.

The prologues, to be dealt with variously in these reflections, begin with what is effectively the prototype in *The Travels of the Three English Brothers* (1607) wherein the skill of the master cook, analogous to that of the writer, is taken as the central conceit. Soon after this, Jonson's prologue to *Epicoene* (1609) uses the analogy extensively as a well-developed figure expanding into the reception of the play to come in terms of taste and delight for a diverse and wilful audience prone to wilfully diverse understanding and appreciation. In 1624, John Fletcher makes a closer analogy between ambitious poetic dramas and elaborate, ornate banquet food in his prologue to *A Wife for a Month*:

> You are welcome Gentlemen, and would our Feast
> Were so well season'd, to please every Guests
> Ingenuous appetites, I hope we shall,
> And their examples may prevaile in all
> (Our noble friends); who writ this, bid me say,
> He had rather dresse, upon a Triumph day,
> My Lord Mayers Feast, and make him Sawces too,
> Sauce for each severall mouth, nay further go,
> He had rather build up those invincible Pyes
> And Castle Custards that afright all our eyes,
> Nay eat 'em all, and their Artillery,
> Than dresse for such a curious company
> One single dish; yet he has pleas'd ye too,
> And you have confest he knew well what to do;
> Be hungry as you were wont to be, and bring
> Sharpe stomacks to the stories he shall sing,
> And he dare yet, he saies, prepare a Table
> Shall make you say well drest, and he well able. (Beaumont and Fletcher
> 1966–85, vol.6, 367)

In the 1630s, Carew, for Davenant in *The Wits*, Suckling in *The Goblins*, and Brome in *The Lovesick Court* make free use of the analogy between theatrical and gustatory taste, all perhaps inspired by Jonson's use of the imagery in his prologues; they were all within his circle of influence, to be sure. As we shall see, Jonson's prologues make comprehensive use of culinary metaphor as well as offering an opportunity to confront an audience with his case for the improved status of the poet. Rhetorical over-ornamentation and over-elaborate culinary excess are also compared in these examples of preliminary matter. After the less than happy reception of *The New Inn* in performance, the poet Cleveland replies to Jonson's 'Ode to himself', including a stanza echoing and enhancing Jonson's prologue imagery with additional reference to banquets (Cleveland 1910, 503). As quoted in the opening epigram, Thomas Carew in 1634, addresses a prologue to 'The Reader' of *The Wits* to be followed by Suckling in his prologue to *The Goblins* (1638). Suckling develops the idea and makes it work for him as an overview of drama, dramatists and dramaturgy, a background against which to set his play in a particular context. Brome uses the device last, in 1639, as a diffident plea for recognition, couched in culinary metaphor. His use of the imagery in the prologue to *The Lovesick Court* is less ambitious than his predecessors' but retains the spirit of the previous prologues and addresses:

> Sometimes at poor mens boards the curious finde
> 'Mongst homely fare, some unexpected dish,
> Which at great Tables they may want and wish:

If in this slight Collation you will binde
Us to believe you'have pleasd your pallats here,
Pray bring your friends w'you next, you know your cheer. (Brome 1658, F2v)

In the first of these prologues identified, Day's (with Rowley and Wilkins) *The Travels of the Three English Brothers* (1607) direct analogy between the role of the dramatist and that of the master cook is encouraged:

Our scene is mantled in the robe of truth,
Yet must we crave, by law of poesy
To give our history an ornament
But equalling this definition, thus:
Who gives a fowl unto his cook to dress
Likewise expects to have a fowl again.
Though in the cook's laborious workmanship
Much may be diminished, somewhat added –
The loss of feathers and the gain of sauce –
Yet in the back surrender of this dish
It is, and may be truely called, the same.
Such are our acts. (Day, Rowley, and Wilkins 1995, *Prologue* 5–16)

The relationship of source material to the finished product – raw poultry in the case of the cook and borrowed narrative in the case of the dramatist – are seen as directly comparable in terms of their subsequent transformation. The implications of the altered state of the materials are suggested as distinctly philosophical ones. The essential notion of the 'raw' as distinct from the 'cooked' directs the auditor or reader to the very heart of what characterises human civilisation. It invites the audience to consider the cooking process as one that is uniquely human and raises humankind above all those animals, so many of which find their selves the raw material. Harvard anthropologist Richard Wrangham, who has done much work on the evolution of cooking and on cooking's influence upon evolution of the human species, considers cooking to have been the single major advance that turned ape *into* human, eons prior to the civilisation of humankind (Wrangham 2009). Claude Lévi-Strauss in his *The Raw and the Cooked*, emphasised the cultural dimensions of cooking to the subsequent development of civilised behaviours in humans over the millennia:

All these customs [...] we must compare and contrast before we can isolate their common features and hope to understand them. They all seem to depend, more or less explicitly, on the contrast between the cooked and the raw, or between nature and culture, the two contrasts being readily confused in linguistic usage. (Lévi-Strauss 1981, 335)

This has been understood to lie behind the essential nature of cookery as a definitive cultural marker: 'Since cooking is an act of mediation, where we transform raw materials into a cooked product, so myths regularly "view culinary operations as

mediatory activities between heaven and earth, life and death, nature and society'"
(Ashley, Hollow, Jones, and Taylor 2004, 29–30). The *cook* is, of course, that
mediator, and one we encounter in early Greek culture through the role of the
mageiros, the 'cook-sacrificer' (see below). In such cultures 'the act of cooking
operates as a symbolic marker between a series of binary oppositions (heaven/
earth, life/death, nature/culture)' (Ashley, Hollow, Jones, and Taylor 2004, 29). So,
for Lévi-Strauss and his followers, cooking marks that transition from 'nature' to
'culture', raw to the cooked, natural to the more sophisticated. Judith Williamson,
in her work on advertisements for cooked products, uses Lévi-Strauss' analysis
and concludes that 'if a culture is to refer to itself, therefore, it can only do so by
the representation of its transformation of nature – it has meaning in terms of what
it has *changed*' (Williamson 1978, 103).

The changed state of the cooked over the raw as outlined by Day's prologue
wittily chooses fowl, almost the only meat source which retains its original name
in English when cooked. From 1066 onwards, 'raw' Anglo-Saxon cows became
'cooked' Norman, noble beef; sheep likewise became mutton, pigs or swine became
pork, and so on. As well as socio-linguistic cultural engineering by a conquering
power, there is a whole process of euphemism at work, of course, which centuries
of usage have efficiently obscured via familiarity. Amusingly, more recent attempts
to market new meats for the domestic table have had advertisers in difficulties
because this sanitising process is not so easy to achieve post-haste. The attempt to
market jointed kangaroo as 'jump-meat' is perhaps one of the more entertainingly
desperate results of the exercise to make 'cuddly', 'cute', or off-beat meat sources
acceptable as food. In this prologue, however, the generic term 'fowl' complicates
the matter nicely in a way which playfully borders on the profound. When fowl
is processed in the kitchen and presented at table, chicken remains chicken,
goose goose, pigeon pigeon, pheasant pheasant, partridge partridge, and so forth:
'it is, and may be truelie cald, the same'. In essence it philosophically predates
Descartes's *Meditations on the First Philosophy in which the Existence of God
and the Real Distinction Between the Soul and the Body of Man are Demonstrated*,
by some thirty or more years. In the *Second Meditation* Descartes proposes:

> Let us take, for example, this piece of wax which has just been taken from the
> hive; it has not yet lost the sweetness of the honey it contained; it still retains
> something of the smell of the flowers from which it was gathered; its colour,
> shape and size are apparent; it is hard, cold, it is tangible; and if you tap it, it
> will emit a sound. [...] But as I am speaking, it is placed near a flame: what
> remained of its taste is dispelled, the smell disappears, its colour changes, it
> loses its shape, it grows bigger, becomes liquid, warms up, one can hardly
> touch it, and, although one taps it, it will no longer make any sound. Does the
> same wax remain after this change? [...] Certainly it could be nothing of all the
> things which I perceived by means of the senses, for everything which fell under
> taste, smell, sight, touch or hearing, is changed, and yet the same wax remains.
> (Descartes 1968, 108–9)

He 'cannot conceive of it in this way without possessing a human mind' (Descartes
1968, 111). Indeed, the nature of the human mind itself is revealed to him by the

translated form of the wax, carrying the suggestion of a state beyond an object's inherent 'flexibility' and 'malleability' (Descartes 1968, 109). Day (Rowley or Wilkins), as befits a witty writer of entertainments rather than a proto-Cartesian philosopher, takes the paradox of the illusory reversibility and crowns it with a delightful metaphysical conceit generated and sustained by linguistic ambiguity.

The extract also prises open another aspect of the creative process, that of writing plays based (almost invariably) upon pre-existing narrative and dramatic sources. For writers of the period, playwriting, like cookery, is essentially an adaptation process, a process of changing raw materials, and an often collaborative one at that. 'Laborious workmanship' translates material from one medium into another ('the loss of feathers and the gain of sauce'), implying a change from a lesser form into a higher one, the raw into the cooked, the prosaic into the poetic, the uncouth into a sophisticated or more civilised format, the better for human consumption. Robert Greene's infamous putdown of 'Shakes-scene' in the previous century, as 'an upstart Crow, beautified with our feathers' (Greene 1592, F1v), lays bare all the resentment of those would-be Macrobian crows wantonly stealing material without acknowledgement. The audacity, however, lies not with an act of theft but in the translation from one state into another, the metamorphosis into a new medium, that of popular drama. That new medium by the 1590s had already revealed its insatiability for fresh material. Talented writers took what already existed and did not devise their own raw materials for a variety of good reasons. They behaved like cooks, in fact. First, it was endorsed by a tradition of already established dramaturgical practice. Sackville and Norton, for example in *Gorboduc*, imitated their classical model, Seneca, in taking a story from distant myth or legend, as Seneca himself had looked to earlier Greek stories for material. Sackville and Norton looked to English pre-history. Preston's *Cambyses* took its story from Heroditus, Peele took *David and Bethsabe* from the Bible. It was common practice, therefore, in the nascent dramatic writings of the sixteenth-century, endorsed by classical precedent, by earlier dramatists, and Aristotle as passed down through the medieval translators and interpreters.

A second reason was clearly the positive advantage of using available ingredients or ingredient material that was a known quantity. An established story had a narrative integrity in its own right and provided a framework at the very least for any translation into another medium or genre. Being well known was an advantage in rendering it more easily understandable to a new audience. A third and equally pragmatic reason was that the dramatists were adding voice and movement to what came from the page, and therein lay the novelty or ingenuity. This equated to a 'gain of sauce' traded off against 'the loss of feathers' by the cook. There was little incentive to be inventive as regards narrative, little need in fact to search for storylines and ideas when there was an abundance of material waiting to be adapted. It was all part and parcel of a particular late sixteenth- and early seventeenth-century re-circulation of texts in many guises. These texts, of course, fell into two main categories of ingredient: the definable, direct, identifiable material on which the writer demonstrably drew; and the more indirect material which derived from an accretion of commonplaces, or ideas created by an indefinable process of mutation in the mind by the subliminal metamorphosis of a lifetime's reading. Literary sources were the whole relevant contents of the writer's mind as he composed. With the exercise of expertise by the writer, these underwent the processes of adaptation, transformation, transmutation from one state into another, to emerge in the new medium of popular drama. All of these narrative sources – poems, chronicles, romances, or history books – were raw ingredients to be transmogrified into a new staged reality. It was undeniably a voracious medium, one with a rapid turnover of material and unstinting demand for new plays, if Henslowe's performance records and receipts for early 1594 are anything to go by. A section of Henslowe's accounts indicate that 18 plays were performed by the Admiral's Men over a typical 13-week period, including seven new plays, averaging one a fortnight over the season (Foakes and Rickert 1961, 26–9). As regards the playwrights' relationship with their source materials, Kiernan Ryan strikes an appropriate metaphor when he reminds us that there is a need to 'respect the inventive agency of the author [...] and see how the texts were actively fashioned out of other texts', but one must be wary of the risk of collapsing the plays 'back into their source materials and generic antecedents, thus mistaking the ingredients for the meal' (Ryan 1999, 8).

As well as suggesting parallels between the handling of the cook's raw materials and the writer's source materials, the underlying conceit of these prologues, which invites audiences to see playwrights as cooks, encourages a broad discussion about the inter-relationship between writers' creativity and cookery. Furthermore, the 'cook' metaphor potentially offers us a contemporary perspective on the very nature of authorship. The creative kinship of cooking to the writing of plays is made in both a positive and negative manner in the late sixteenth and early seventeenth centuries. Stephen Gosson in *The Schoole of Abuse*, 'conteining a plesaunt invective against Poets, Pipers, Plaiers, Jesters and such like Caterpillers of the commonwealth', is keen to 'liken Poetes to Cookes, the pleasures of the one winnes the body from labor, and conquereth the sense; the allurement of the other drawes the mind from virtue, and confoundeth wit' (Gosson 1579, A4v). Dangerously for the polemical Gosson, the comparison would appear, ironically, to be an equivocal one rather than a clinching rhetorical device to distinguish between two poles of praise and condemnation. 'Cookes did never shew more craft in their junckets to vanquish the taste [...] then Poets in Theaters to wound the conscience' (Gosson 1579, B6v). The success of the former, however, would seem to imply that of the latter in making moral points to prick a conscience; that would be part of the role of the true poet for Gosson, and for Sir Philip Sidney in due course. On the poets' (and cooks') side of the analogy, we have the aforementioned endorsement of Carew (above) that 'Poets are Cooks', plus that of Jonson in the introductory material for *Neptune's Triumph*, that 'a good poet differs nothing at all from the master-cook [...] Either's art is the wisdom of the mind' (Jonson 1981– 82, *Prologue* 24–32). Significantly, both cook and dramatist are professionals in the business of producing items of innate ephemerality; performances or meals are made to be seen, or heard/eaten, then they are gone until the next time the text or recipe evoke them into being. To equate an acting text to a recipe is not an entirely satisfactory analogy, but it is, nonetheless, a contemporary comparison invoked by the cook Robert May for his purposes in the seventeenth century (see below), and implicit in the figures composed by the writers of these dramatic prologues. The solution, nonetheless, to rendering the ephemeral in some way, shape, or form concrete is in part found by the printing of a play text or a recipe. For some dramatists, the 'recipe' might perhaps have lain at one remove, in texts such as Aristotle's *Ars Poetica* rather than individual quartos, but the best of dramatists tended to be wilfully iconoclastic about such books of rules.

The reputation of English cooks in the period is a somewhat mixed one, but the esteem reserved for the best of them meant that the comparison was not necessarily an unflattering one for the playhouses' writers. A general, social fixation with food and eating seemed to gain the English (and specifically their *master cooks*) a high reputation in the sixteenth and seventeenth centuries at home and even abroad. English eating, cooking, and hospitality in general were highly regarded. In *An Itinerary* (1617) Fynes Moryson wrote:

> In generall the art of Cookery is much esteemed in England, neither doe any sooner find a Master than men of that profession, and howsoever they are most esteemed which for all kinds are most exquisite in that Art. (Moryson 1617, 150)

William Harrison in his 'Description of England' from Holinshed's *Chronicles* (1587) noted with pride that English 'tables are oftentimes more plentifully garnished than those of other nations' and that 'in number of dishes and change of meat the nobility of England do most exceed' (Holinshed 1587, 132). Clearly, in England in both the sixteenth and seventeenth –centuries, the quality and quantity of cooked food could, among the higher echelons of society at least, be sources of national pride. This reputation of cooks in England and their status is more difficult to square with some of the literary representations and references to their cooking practices. The dramatic representations in contemporary and classical plays, to be dealt with in more detail below, assign cooks more morally ambiguous roles, show them inclined to dubious culinary practices, and suggest associations with infernal kitchens. There are many figurative allusions to the poor quality of their products and the corners that cooks habitually cut in bringing food to the table. An ambiguity of this sort hangs over the contemporary description of Cardinal Wolsey's presumptuous master cook, for example: 'in his private kitchen he had a master cook who went daily in damask, satin or velvet with a chain of gold about his neck' (Strong 2002, 89). Given age-old sumptuary restrictions governing status and the wearing of opulent fabrics, plus the cost of such things, a cook in his daily wear being seen so attired seems quite remarkable evidence of status. It may well be intended, however, as both anti-Wolsey exaggeration and outraged ridicule of the cook's pretensions in the cardinal's service. Adopting such socially transgressive costume would certainly have found him deeply in contravention of the Elizabethan Sumptuary Laws in the final quarter of the century. In comparison, even at the end of the century, Shakespeare's steward Malvolio in *Twelfth Night* (household superior to a master cook) could only conceive of branched velvet gowns and rich jewels about his neck in his wildest fantasies.

A fascination with cookery and the stagey etiquette of dining is clear from the succession of printed books on the subject over the period. *A Proper new Book of Cookerie*, 1575; T. Dawson's *Good Huwife's Jewell, parts one and two*, 1584 and 1585, *The Treasurie of Commodious Conceites*, 1584 (enlarged 1596); *Widowe's Treasure*, 1585; *The Good Huswife's handmaide for the Kitchen*, 1588; and a second edition of Dawson in 1596 cover some of the sixteenth-century examples. As for the first part of the seventeenth century, Sir Hugh Platt's *Delightes for Ladies* was first published in 1605, and Gervase Markham's *The English Huswife* went through five editions between 1615 and 1649. All of these publications lead to the singular, self-fashioning achievement of Robert May and his seventeenth-century publication of *The Accomplisht Cook*. Despite its publication date, *The Accomplisht Cook* was a project emerging from the late sixteenth and early seventeenth centuries. It was conceived ante-bellum but only realised at the Restoration when the prevailing asceticism of the Commonwealth period was relaxed and sybaritic pleasures offered by fine cookery were more sympathetically received by the new regime. Born in 1588, Robert May served his apprenticeship under his father, a master cook, and took further tuition in France until, as a master cook in his own right in 1609, he went forth to cook for several aristocratic households to great acclaim over a 55-year career. *The Accomplisht Cook* is a landmark folio publication in that it foregrounds the master cook as author, not only of his own store of recipes but also of his own destiny: 'it hath been my ambition, that you should be sensible of my Proficiency of Endeavours in this Art' (May 1665, A4r). The work is prefaced by a biography, 'A short Narrative of some Passages of the Authors Life' in pursuit of the 'Art of Cookery'. Projection of the status of English cookery and cooks is the motivation of his publication: 'that I might give a testimony to my Countrey of the laudableness of our Profession' (May 1665, A4r–A4v). Those publications which had gone before he holds as 'empty and unprofitable treatises, of as little use as some Niggards Kitchen, which the Reader in respect of the confusion of the method, or barrenness of those Authors experience, hath rather been puzzled then profited by' (May 1665, A5r). The biography places his roots in the late years of the sixteenth century, when his experience accumulated in a variety of placements until he returned to his father's side as one of five under-cooks in the Dormer household. These were the 'Golden Days wherein were practised the Triumphs and Trophies of Cookery' (May 1665, A6v). Branching out under his own name, he served 12 different aristocratic and bourgeois masters and mistresses without any apparent gaps in employment until the Restoration, when he was able to publish the book in question at last. The publication ran to five editions over the following 20 years. He not only exemplifies a representative English cook of high reputation in the late sixteenth and early seventeenth centuries but also provides us with a cross-over figure of the cook as writer, a writer to whom (albeit mediocre) poets were moved to write tributes. The folio's prefatory material echoes our theatrical examples in metaphor and ambition. James Parry finds much to praise in May's skills as a cook:

[…] as Art in Cookery
Which of the Mathematicks doth pertake,
Geometry proportions when they bake.
Who can in paste erect (of finest flour)
A compleat Fort, a Castle, or a Tower.
A City Custard doth so subtly wind.
That should Truth seek, she'd scarce all corners find;
Platforms of Sconces, that might soldiers teach,
To fortifie by works as well as Preach.
I'le say no more; for as I am a sinner,
I've wrought my self a stomach to a dinner.
Inviting Poets not to tantalize
But feast, (not surfeit) here their Fantasies. (May 1665, B1r)

John Town provides him with the following tribute invoking the spirits of two dead prologue writers from the plays, beginning:

See here's a Book set forth with such things in't
As former Ages never saw in print;
Something I'de write in praise on't, but the Pen,
Of famous Cleaveland, or renowned Ben,
If unintomb'd might give this Book its due,
By their high strains, and keep it always new. [...] (May 1665, B1r)

It should not be forgotten, when considering this comparison between cooks and playwrights, that the two activities (cookery and the production of plays) are, by their natures, collaborative enterprises to a significant extent. The collaboration in the context of creating plays could begin even at the stage of inception:

It has been estimated that almost half of the plays written for the public theatres were of joint authorship. […] Collaboration may have evolved as a means of throwing plays together in a hurry, but at its best it could act as an imaginative stimulus, a pooling of diverse talents conducive to a wider range of dramatic style than individual authors might have achieved on their own. (Wells 2006, 25–7)

So too would be the practice in the bigger kitchens of the period (as outlined below). As an example of the playmaking practices of the time, is hard not to admire the prodigious output and dogged productivity of Thomas Heywood successfully spanning 35 years or more of changing tastes and fashions. His talents were up for hire, and he was promiscuous as well as successful in his professional career. If, as he claimed, he was involved in the creation of 220 plays (as the 'main finger', if nothing else) alongside various other forms of pageant along the way, Heywood represents a prolific, pragmatic and practical breed of writer, versatile and sensitive to the vagaries of popular taste and, above all, always happy to collaborate with others. Jonson was another playwright happy to collaborate at times in his career but, in *Volpone* he makes a point of stating that he

Fully penned it
From his own hand, without a coadjutor,
Novice, journeyman, or tutor. (Jonson 1981–82, *Prologue* 16–19)

This provides us with four levels of collaboration, which are helpfully glossed by Wells, as follows:

Those four nouns usefully define a range of the roles that a collaborator might enact. A coadjutor would be an equal collaborator, a novice a kind of apprentice, a journeyman a hack brought in perhaps to supply a comic subplot, and a tutor a master craftsman guiding a novice. (Wells 2006, 26)

Stephen Orgel has summed up the implications, extent, and nature of this collaborative process by means of which so many of the plays were created:

The company commissioned the play, usually stipulated the subject, often provided the plot, often parcelled it out, scene by scene, to several playwrights. The text thus produced was a working model which the company then revised as seemed appropriate [...] the text belonged to the company, and the authority represented by the text – I am talking now about the *performing* text – is that of the company, the owners, not that of the playwright, the author. (Orgel 1981, 3)

If plays were often akin to group conceptions appearing to de-centre a single author, the metaphor of the cook in a kitchen is particularly intriguing with its hierarchy of operatives under a head chef. Playhouses needed not only writers to co-operate but also the collaboration of players to enact the play texts, plus wardrobe and property staff, musicians, scriveners, stage-hands, and so on, in a similar vein to the kitchen. In *Feast: A History of Grand Eating*, Roy Strong reproduces George Cavendish's contemporary account of Cardinal Wolsey's kitchen structure and manifest of human resources:

He had in the hall-kitchen two clerks of his kitchen, a clerk-controller, a surveyor of the dresser, a clerk of his spicery. Also in his hall-kitchen he had two master cooks and twelve other labourers and children, as they called them; a yeoman of his scullery, with two others in his silver scullery; two yeoman of his pantry and two grooms. Now in his private kitchen he had a master cook who went daily in damask, satin or velvet with a chain of gold about his neck; and two grooms with six labourers and children to serve the place; in the Larder there, a yeoman and a groom; in the Scalding house, a yeoman and two grooms; in the Scullery there, two persons; in the Buttery, two yeomen and two grooms, and two pages; and in the Ewery likewise; in the Cellar three yeomen, two grooms and two pages. (Strong 2002, 89–90)

When Henry VIII in due course took over another of Wolsey's properties at Hampton Court, he had the Lord Steward's department staffed 'by up to two hundred people who ranged from expert cooks to seven small boys employed to turn spits. In the Great Kitchen, under the Master Cook, there were approximately twelve other cooks and a dozen or so assistants. Each of the subsidiary kitchens was under the control of a serjeant who was assisted by up to ten others' (Wigg 1991, 5).

The system persists to this day, of course, with head chef, second chefs, sous chefs, third chefs, commis chefs, kitchen porters, et al. Nonetheless, at the pinnacle of all the creative activity, there exists a space for one 'author' possessed of a singular talent, one master cook as creator-in-chief, a motivator of a team but who is a focal point and is publicly known, indeed renowned, enough to attract the paying customer, patron, or employer. There clearly exists a tension, not surprisingly, between the need for collaboration at a variety of levels and egotistical anxieties about the status of the lead creator of spectacles. It was Jonson, Orgel contends, who best articulated as well as represented this at the time. He succeeded in 'suppressing the theatrical production [...] and replaced it with an independent, printed text which he consistently refers to, moreover, not as a play but as a poem' (Orgel 1981, 4). He took the step of transforming theatrical script to literary text: 'in preparing the play for publication, Jonson took control of the text; he replaced his collaborator's scenes with ones of his own, and added a good deal of new material' (Orgel 1981, 4). With the innovative step of collating and editing his 'works' in folio, the playmaker progressed to the level of dramatic poet with eyes to contemporary reward and the acclaim of posterity. Stallybrass and White cite Jonson as the key to understanding the movement towards the concept, or a self-projection, of the writer as author, contributing 'significantly to the construction of the domain of "authorship" in the period' (Stallybrass and White 1986, 66).

This debate over the relative status attached to the poet (or aspirant, ambitious cook) as creative artist against that of the skilful artisan or craft worker exemplified in Jonson's anxiety, invites an analogy with the experience of the fine artist in the earlier part of the Renaissance across Europe. Both Ben Jonson and Robert May envisaged their respective projects in folio as monuments to their artistic aspiration and achievement. The case had already been made for fine artists in the years up to 1550, when Giorgio Vasari's *The Lives of the most eminent Italian Architects, Painters and Sculptors* was published and ultimately became the defining text in the debate. The change in perception as to the relative standings of practitioners of the liberal arts and their social position as artists was not a uniform and linear projection. At different times in different places in Europe, artists had already been deemed great, achieved greatness, or had greatness thrust upon them by chroniclers, customers, or patrons. As early as 1400, Cennino Cennini made the case in his treatise on art that a transformation was already being made from the craft worker to that of the artist with an identity. The transition in status from artisan to artist was clearly made for sixteenth-century fine artists like Raphael, Michelangelo, and Titian, in Italy at least. A more apposite example for the purposes of comparison with English professional dramatists and cooks is perhaps Albrecht Durer. With his bold self-portraiture, monogrammed, branded signings of his works, deliberate reproducibility, and self promotion he achieved an elevation in status beyond that of journeyman – without the help of Vasari's *Lives* and without the advantages of southern European Church or state patronage. The uncertainty as to the relative merits of the artist as against the artisan had always hinged on the part played by *ingegno* in true artistry, and finds echoes in both the May and Jonson projects.

Jonson clearly saw a useful exemplary link between his own art and that of the cook by his persistent use of culinary metaphor in the prologues and elsewhere within his plays. It is clear from the following example (so pertinent that he used it twice), in the cancelled masque *Neptune's Triumph* from 1624 and in *The Staple of News*:

> A master cook! Why he's the man o' men,
> For a professor! He designs, he draws,
> He paints, he carves, he builds, he fortifies,
> Makes citadels of curious fowl and fish. (Jonson 1981–82, IV.ii.19–22)

The dramatist's aspiration to poet, to move from something perceived as craft worker (i.e. play*wright*, or play*maker*) to dramatic poet is clearly one that Jonson felt keenly. Admittedly, it was not universally felt; hence the tilting at Jonson's pretentiousness in collecting and publishing his works voiced by some minor satirists and epigrammatists at the time. It was still being teasingly alluded to 30 years later by Suckling, for example, in 'A Session of the Poets' from his *Fragmenta Aurea* collection:

> The first that broke silence was good old Ben,
> Prepared before with canary wine,
> And he told them plainly he deserved the bays
> For his were called works, where others were but plays. (Suckling 1971, vol. 1.
> 12–15)

In 1598, John Florio's Italian-English dictionary glossed the crucial term *ingegno* as 'wit, arte, skill, knowledge'; he implied inventiveness and ingenuity on the part of an *ingegnoso*, one who was 'wittie, ingenious [and] full of invention' (Florio 1598, 181). Vasari (after others such as Leon Battista Alberti) took the Italian word as representing that which could not be taught and could not be acquired, denied to all but the few touched by this particular form of genius, as it became commonly translated in foreign texts. It also touches upon that related notion of the artist as an individual endowed with *ingegno* as distinct from those creatures of collaboration and co-operation with assistants in workshops or guilds of association. The cult of the subjectivity of the artist grew from this and the role of biography (as used by Alberti and then Vasari) in proposing the special qualities and experiences of a singularly endowed individual clearly finds its counterpart in the conscious inclusion of Robert May's life story in *The Accomplisht Cook*.

Another aspect of the debate over the status of playwright as poet, the transformer of the prosaic into the poetic, is one which others of the prologues direct us to next. After the less than happy reception of Jonson's *The New Inn* in performance, the poet Cleveland replied to Jonson's 'Ode to himself', including a stanza echoing and enhancing Jonson's prologue imagery with further reference to banquets. He directs the auditor to look to the ancient Greek models and Menander in particular as classical endorsement:

But if thou make thy feasts
For the high-relish'd guests,
And that a cloud of shadows shall break in,
It were almost a sin
To think that thou shouldst equally delight
Each several appetite;
Though Art and Nature strive
Thy banquets to contrive:
Thou art our whole Menander, and dost look
Like the old Greek; think, then, but on his Cook. (Cleveland 1910, 503)

Not that there exist many examples, but 'the best preserved plays of Menander all present cooks' (Scodel 1993,161), and by reputation, Menander's cooks were loquacious, boastful, and users of grandiose language. On stage they claimed magical powers, put down any rivals, itemised lists of food both real and fantastical, and were often portrayed as working in, or having just worked in, a hot kitchen; R. Scodel points out that 'As a character, this type of cook appears first in [Menandrian] Middle Comedy' (1993, 162). This stage representation of the cook occurred within a culturally specific but highly relevant context, to do with the role of the Greek *mageiros*: 'In the socio-cultural reality from the fifth-century BC onward, the different operations of the sacrifice are undertaken by one person, the *mageiros*, the butcher-cook-sacrificer' (Detienne and Vernant 1989, 11). This notion of a cook-sacrificer could be said to hover behind the prologue to *The Travels of the Three English Brothers*, wherein a residual notion of sacrifice hangs upon the process of offering up something transformed and precious. The ritual, mystic, and quasi-religious associations of the role of cook-sacrificer were ones which gradually merged with the artisan qualities of the cook and co-existed from the Greeks onwards. According to J. C. B. Lowe, seven 'scenes of Plautus's plays in which cooks appear [demonstrate that] Plautus's cooks show both Greek and Roman characteristics in differing degrees' (1985, 85). There came about an inter-relationship between Greek *mageiros* and the Roman *coquus* who more often, in real life, was an ordinary household slave with a particular skill in the kitchen. It was, in any case, more likely for Renaissance writers to have drawn their conclusions about cooks from their knowledge of Plautus, inheritor of the raw materials of Menandrian comic tropes and styles. His influence upon the playwrights of the late sixteenth and early seventeenth centuries enabled Menandrian scraps to be worked up into more substantial fare. Nonetheless, 'no-one doubts that Plautus's cooks are in some sense the heirs of the *mageiroi* of Greek comedy [representing] the combination of ritual and culinary functions which attached to the person of the *mageiros*, professional sacrificer as well as butcher and cook' (Lowe 1985, 72–3). The blended roles of cook and sacrificer, along with the accumulated character traits, were such that cooks became 'a stock character of comedy, with certain conventional characteristics, chief among which are pretentiousness and loquacity [of one who] claims to be an expert and is full of self-importance' (Lowe 1985, 74–5).

Intriguingly, Sir Philip Sidney's reflections in *The Defence of Poesy* upon the definition of the word 'poet' and the derivation of the term betrays some overlap with the respective roles of the cook as *coquus* and as the *mageiros* of Greek comedy:

> Among the Romans a poet was called *vates* which is as much as a diviner, foreseer, or prophet, as by his conjoined words *vaticinium* and *vaticinari* is manifest: so heavenly a title did that excellent people bestow upon this heart-ravishing knowledge [...] But now let us see how the Greeks named it, and how they deemed it. The Greeks called him a 'poet', which name hath, as the most excellent, gone through other languages. It cometh of this word *poiein*, which is, to make: wherein I know not whether by luck or wisdom, we Englishmen have met with the Greeks in calling him a maker. (Sidney 1989, 214–15)

Sidney's *vates* corresponds in some degree to the ritual sacrificer, the shamanic *mageiros*, and the 'maker' to the crafty cook, with craft to be read in both senses of the word. In this context, the suggestion that, in his turn, 'Plato uses the *mageiros* as a simile for the dialectician who must cut up a *logos* correctly' (Scodel 1993, 170) places the cook-sacrificer alongside the poet as a supreme handler of language, not just a plausible and entertaining loudmouth. It also directly revisits an aspect of the debate (above) about the status of the dramatist as poet, or as playwright or play maker.

The second implication of the reference to Menander and the 'old Greeks' in Cleveland's reply to Jonson's *Ode to Himself*, is that cooks for the literary fraternity bear some imprint of their classical precedents and their characteristics were known ones. 'Plautus has six cooks in his corpus' (Scodel 1993, 161), who demonstrate the stock qualities of the Greek comic *mageiros* to which are added, on occasion, concerns about pay, a propensity for theft, a talent for scurrilous abuse, and occasional physical violence, such that eventually in Plautine comedy 'a new comic stereotype replaced that of the *mageiros* of Greek comedy (Lowe 1985, 102). This type of cook was a 'very frequent visitor to the stage. [...] The cook is a fixed type [who] is ridiculously self-important; he claims a noble craft with great traditions, pedantically lecturing his employer, and imparting the mysteries of his art [...] is pompous, boring, nosy, often a thief and a kvetch' (Scodel 1993, 161). Furthermore, he operates within his world of the kitchen, an exclusive domain wherein 'his high ambition leads to a greater elaboration than straightforward "feasting". This expands the attention paid to provisioning, the work of the kitchen, and elaboration at table' (Wilkins 2001, 372). All in all, a Greek comic cook in his world sounds very like a working playwright in his.

Given these known characteristics, what examples do we have of cooks on stage in sixteenth- and early seventeenth-century plays, and to what extent do they reflect the classical precedent of 'the old Greeks' highlighted in Cleveland's ode? A couple of late sixteenth-century examples are brief, and not in comedies: Collen the cook is required on stage with detailed directions for inclusion in *Alphonsus, Emperor of Germany* (1594), replete with 'a gammon of raw bacon and links or puddings in a platter' (Chapman 1961, III.i.132SD). He says nothing. The eponymous hero appears 'like a cook' in the final act of Shakespeare's *Titus Andronicus* (1594). Titus as sacrificer could be argued as a motif implied by the assumption of cook's guise in the final section of the play, as he wields his knife to devastating effect in the deaths of daughter Lavinia and Empress Tamora, having despatched and butchered the latter's two sons in the high sacrificial style of a *mageiros* in the previous scene. Three more substantial examples from the period of the prologues that concern us here do, however, occur in *The Old Law* (Middleton, 1618), Fletcher's *The Bloody Brother, The Tragedy of Rollo* (1619), and in *A New Way to Pay Old Debts* by Massinger in 1621. Two cooks in comedies, and one from a tragedy. In Middleton's *The Old Law*, we are actually transported to an ancient Greek setting, and early in the play we are introduced to key members of the Master's household (cook, butler, tailor, bailiff) who are all faced with the sack. The cook is reasonably eloquent and argues for his own indispensability ('Marry Sir, a cook, I know your mastership cannot be without', Middleton 1982, II.i), but to no avail. He does not come across as particularly boastful, however, and in the ensuing stratagems he more often than not defers to the butler's counsel. In the third act he again appears as part of the package of redundant retainers who embark on the butler's scheme to cozen rich old widows into brief marriages. By the end of the play they have been out-tricked, out-talked, and out-thought by the clown, Gnothos, and ultimately outwitted as a group in a fifth-act dénouement. Despite Greek references littered throughout their below-stairs dialogue, and lively repartee between him and his household companions, the cook figure of Menandrian or Plautine Comedy is hard to discern in Middleton's representation of a cook on stage here.

Fletcher's *The Bloody Brother, The Tragedy of Rollo* (1619) contains a significant antagonist in the master cook who first appears in the second act along with his household peers, the butler, pantler, and yeoman of the cellar who all defer to him. The cook is hot from the kitchen, combining associations both of Vulcan and Satan, and is a prodigious drinker. He turns out to be a boaster in praise of his own skills, and ultimately proves corruptible. His bragging portrays him as an entertainer, a summoner-up of action, not unlike a dramatic writer of masques in fact:

> Ile make yee pigs speak French at table, and a fat Swan
> Come sailing out of England with a challenge,
> Ile make yee a dish of Calves feet dance the Canaries,
> And a consort of cram'd Capons fiddle to em.
> A Calves head speak an Oracle, and a dozen of Larkes
> Rise from the dish, and sing all supper time […]
> Arion on a Dolphin playing Lachrimae,
> And brave King Herring with his oyl and onion
> Crownd with leomon pill, his way prepar'd
> With his strong guard of pilchers […]
> If you'l have the pastie speak, 'tis in my power. (Beaumont and Fletcher 1966–
> 85, II.ii.10–15, 22–25, 40)

He talks of a 'sacrifice' to Bacchus at his 'altar', where the vintner will kneel and offer 'incense to his Deity' (Beaumont and Fletcher 1966–85, II.ii.34, 38). The second phase of this extended domestic scene has the cook and his companions suborned to poison the meats at a banquet ostensibly for reconciliation between the two bloody brothers of the title. The cook envisages it thus:

> my finger slipps a little
> Downe drops a dose, I stirre him with my ladle,
> And there's a dish for a Duke [...]
> Here stands a bak't meate, he wants a little seasoning,
> A foolish mistake, my spice-boxe gentlemen,
> And put in some of this, the matters ended. (Beaumont and Fletcher 1966–85, II.ii.157–62)

When all comes to light, the staff are led off to execution in the third act, the eloquent cook leading them all in facing death bravely, literally with a song on their lips: 'Yet but looke on the master Cook / The glory of the kitchin' (Beaumont and Fletcher 1966–85, III.ii.67–8). In addition to some recognisable elements of the Menandrian and Plautine comedic cook in Fletcher's character, there is, more pertinently, a contemporary resonance to the cook as a poisoner. In 1616, Sir Thomas Overbury was murdered by cook Richard Weston, who was found guilty and executed for administering poison in broth possibly at his mistress's request (Hensman 1974, vol. 2 265).

A New Way to Pay Old Debts (Massinger, 1621) provides our final staged example of an early seventeenth-century comic cook. In the *Dramatis Personae* he is granted a name, Furnace, appropriate to his role in the kitchen, redolent once again of Vulcan and hellfire and shorthand for his displays of the choleric humour. With his peers and with his betters he maintains a free-spoken manner, takes the initiative in arguing his corner, and is impeccably loyal to his employer, a rich widow who pines on a disappointing diet of *panada* or water gruel despite the cook's attempts to tempt her. The cook resents the fact that his best offerings are diverted into the stomach of insatiate Justice Greedy. His witty putdowns of Greedy in the following scenes are testament to the cook's wit and quickness of thought. He later significantly succeeds as the maker of a magically restorative elixir. As the play progresses, he becomes party to the twists and turns of the main plot and often appears above stairs as a crafty servant always in support of the family of his employer (another Plautine comedy staple). He is an essential part of the denouement and the happy resolution of the play as a whole. Despite some degree of eloquence in common (leaving aside Collen), it is only with this final example that a stage cook bears substantial hallmarks of classical precedent.

Any cook, whether staged or real, prepares meals to be presented, consumed, and judged; so too the playwright sets forth a play to an audience and an uncertain reception. Ubiquitous in these prologues is the metaphor of gustatory and literary 'taste', figuratively allied with tasting and tastiness. This focuses upon the potential parallels between the 'appetite', the application of the 'palate', and the way in which an audience reacts with good or bad 'taste' to the play to come or the play's first run of performances. It coincides with an explicit evocation of Epicurus and his apostolic epicures with their epicurean appetites in Suckling's *The Goblins* in 1638 and Carew, for Davenant, in *The Wits*, earlier in 1634.

Wit in a prologue, poets justly may
Stile a new imposition on a play.
When Shakespeare, Beaumont, Fletcher rul'd the stage,
There scarce were ten good palates in the age;
More curious cooks than guests; for men would eat
Most heartily of any kind of meat.
And then what strange variety ! each play
A feast for Epicures ! and that, each day.
But mark how oddly it is come about,
And how unluckily it now falls out;
The palates are grown high, number increas'd,
And there wants that which should make up the feast;
And yet y'are so unconsionable, you'd have
Forsooth of late, that which they never gave;
Banquets before and after. (Suckling 1971, vol. 2 *Prologue* 1–15)

It hath been said of old, that plays are feasts,
Poets the cooks, and the spectators guests,
The actors waiters: from this simile
Some have deriv'd an unsafe liberty,
To use their judgments as their tastes; which choose,
Without controul, this dish, and that refuse.
But Wit allows not this large privilege;
Either you must confess, or feel its edge:
Nor shall you make a current inference,
If you transfer your reason to your sense.
Things are distinct, and must the same appear
To every piercing eye, or well-tun'd ear.
Though sweets with your's, sharps best with my taste meet,
Both must agree this meat's or sharp or sweet:
But if I scent a stench or a perfume,
Whilst you smell nought at all, I may presume
You have that sense imperfect: so you may
Affect a merry, sad, or humourous play.
If, though the kind distaste or please, the good
And bad be by your judgment understood:
But if, as in this play, where with delight
I feast my *epicurean appetite*
With relishes so curious, as dispense
The utmost pleasure to the ravish'd sense,
You should profess that you can nothing meet
That hits your taste either with sharp or sweet,
But cry out, 'Tis insipid; your bold tongue
May do it's master, not the author, wrong;
For men of better palate will, by it,
Take the just elevation of your wit. (Davenant 1968, vol. 2 165–94)

Persistent scholarly and popular misinterpretation of the true nature of Epicurus's writings led to epicurism equating to a gourmand tendency at table in pursuit of pleasure. This was a misreading of Epicurus's advocacy of reliance upon the senses, but the currency of it stuck. Life's goal for Epicurus may well have been happiness in tranquillity, but the route was to apply rule, or *ratio*, to the passions and the appetite rather than to indulge a human tendency to the hedonism and self-gratification attributed to his followers by subsequent interpreters. (Ironically, if writers had had access to his actual works, postulating the structure of the world as a series of combinations of atoms, then another potentially useful analogy of play-writing in relation to source material would have been there for the taking.) The typical view that emerged is encapsulated in Chaucer's take on epicureans in his Prologue to *The Canterbury Tales*. The Franklin displays all the relevant signs of the serial epicure:

> Wel loved he by the morwe a sop in wyn
> To liven in delyt was ever his wone,
> For he was Epicurus owne sone [...]
> His breed, his ale, was alwey after oon;
> A better envyned man was no-wher noon.
> With oute bake mete was never his hous,
> Of fish and flesh, and that so plenteuous
> It snowed in his hous of mete and drinke
> Of alle deyntees that men coude thinke.
> After the sundry sesons of the yeer
> So chaunged he his mete and his soper [...]
> Wo was his cook, but if his sauces were
> Poynaunt and sharp, and redy al his gere. (Chaucer 1962, 423)

By the Renaissance, the works of Epicurus were still misrepresented and misunderstood to be synonymous with hedonism and gluttony in general. Epicurism is still associated with these indulgences in the early seventeenth century, in Jonson's *The Alchemist* and *Volpone* for example. These seventeenth-century prologues, however, imply a degree of fastidiousness in the epicure, suggesting a redeeming sense of refinement and discernment on the part of those of an epicurean bent. It is a significant shift towards the modern usage of the term generally, with a shift from gourmand to gourmet in the epicure.

The playwrights' view of any given audience or audiences in general clearly emerges within the prologues. The nature of, and the discernment shown by, audiences can be seen as a perennial source of frustration for the dramatists. They attempt to flatter, but when rebuffed by a poor reception, the humiliation sparks impotent hostility couched in language redolent of the most humble plea to the patrons of an earlier age as expressed in dedications aplenty, or vindictive criticism via analogy. As Stallybrass and White note, 'Again and again, Jonson defines the true position of the playwright as that of the poet, and the poet as that of the classical isolated judge standing in opposition to the vulgar throng' (1986, 66–7). This is made most clear in Jonson's prologues and supplementary materials. As these reflections have progressed, Jonson seems to emerge more and more as a *nexus* anchoring a web of influence in this business of culinary metaphor. The writers of the prologues and associated material are variously contemporaries, companions, collaborators, and, in Brome's case, his manservant and protégé. Jonson was, of course, no stranger to the dining table and the food and drink thereon; he was far from abstemious as an eater or drinker, such that he engrossed to just short of 20 stones in his latter years (Miles 1986, 210). Thus, we end with Jonson and his use of culinary metaphor in two of the prologues to his plays *Epicoene* and *The New Inn*. The first, a boys' company play, fell foul of the taste of the upper tier of London society and the sense of injustice flavours the prologue:

> But in this age a sect of writers are,
> That only for particular likings care
> And will taste nothing that is popular.
> With such we mingle neither brains nor breasts;
> Our wishes, like to those make public feasts,
> Are not to please the cook's tastes but the guests'.
> Yet if those cunning palates hither come,
> They shall find guests' entreaty and good room;
> And though all relish not, sure there will be some
> That when they leave their seats, shall make'em say,
> Who wrote that piece could so have wrote a play,
> But that he knew this was the better way.
> For to present all custard or all tart
> And have no other meats to bear a part,
> Or want bread and salt, were but coarse art.
> The Poet prays you then with better thought
> To sit, and when his cates are all in brought,
> Though there be none far fet, there will dear-bought
> Be fit for ladies, some for lords, knights, squires,
> Some for your waiting-wench, and city-wires,
> Some for your men, and daughters of Whitefriars.
> Nor is it only while you keep your seat
> Here that his feast will last, but you shall eat
> A week at ord'naries on his broken meat [...] (Jonson 1981–82, *Prologue* 4–27)

The poet-as-cook metaphor is well worked into the whole prologue and allows Jonson to make his point about the status of the poet seven years before his publication of the *Works*. Much of relevance had happened in the intervening 20 years before his next culinary prologue, to *The New Inn*. It followed Jonson's return to the stage with *The Staple of News* after a deliberate ten-year absence from 'the loathed stage' (Jonson, 'Ode to Himself', 11). Jonson had been Poet Laureate since 1616 and had had his folio published the same year, 'an incalculable contribution to the raising of drama's status in England' (Miles 1986, 171) but, notwithstanding, *The New Inn* was badly received and hissed off the stage at

Blackfriars. The prologue we have left to us reflects Jonson's reaction to the experience, along with the 'Ode to Himself', and the various replies to that ode, such as Cleveland's already dealt with above:

> You are welcome, welcome all to the New Inn:
> Though the old house, we hope our cheer will win
> Your acceptation: we have the same cook
> Still, and the fat, who says, you shall not look
> Long for your bill of fare, but every dish
> Be serv'd in i' the time, and to your wish:
> If any thing be set to a wrong taste,
> 'Tis not the meat there, but the mouth's displaced,
> Remove but that sick palate, all is well.
> For this the more secure dresser bade me tell,
> Nothing more hurts just meetings, than a crowd;
> Or, when the expectation's grown too loud:
> That the nice stomach would have this or that,
> And being ask'd or urged, it knows not what,
> When sharp or sweet, have been too much a feast,
> And both outlived the palate of the guest.
> Beware to bring such appetites to the stage,
> They do confess a weak, sick, queasy age;
> And a shrewd grudging too of ignorance,
> When clothes and faces 'bove the men advance:
> Hear for your health, then, but at any hand,
> Before you judge, vouchsafe to understand,
> Concoct, digest: if then, it do not hit,
> Some are in a consumption of wit,
> Deep he dares say, he will not think, that all -
> For hectics are not epidemical. (Jonson 1981–82, *Prologue* 1–26)

Behind each and every one of these prologues lies a well-developed sense of the kinship between the invention and exciting novelty of the theatrical world and the potential of the best kitchens to create in a similar vein. Jonson made it explicit in *Neptune's Triumph* and again in *The Staple of News*:

> A master cook! Why he's the man o' men,
> For a professor ! He designs, he draws,
> He paints, he carves, he builds, he fortifies,
> Makes citadels of curious fowl and fish. [...] (Jonson 1981–82, IV.ii.19–22)

The image conjured is one of a veritable Leonardo da Vinci, a deliberately vainglorious, comically bathetic evocation of the Renaissance polymath endowed with *ingegno* in superabundance. All of the prologue writers adopt the guise and borrow the characteristics of the eloquent and boastful cook of classical comedy and the renowned contemporary English chefs in order to make a plea for recognition and reward. The cook and the playwriting poet are both dealers in illusion, taking materials from one medium and translating them into another, performing a bravura act of metamorphosis transforming an original into a facsimile in another form. They are masters of the ephemeral and are able to transmogrify ingredient matter in transcendental fashion like a *magus*, or the quasi-religious *mageiros*, or *vates*. Knowing the effectiveness of comedy to make a point, these playwrights employ the poet-as-cook motif and the associated figurative panoply in persistently wry manner; that organ of taste, the tongue, always well ensconced in cheek. The depiction of Jonson's master cook as Renaissance man, Fletcher's Master Cook ('If you'll have the pastie speak, 'tis in my power' *The Bloody Brother*, Beaumont and Fletcher 1966–85, II.ii.40), and all of the other users of the metaphor discussed employ the device to express shared anxieties about their subjectivity, their status, and the reception of their fare. In Shakespeare's *The Tempest*, the writer's putative *alter ego* wields his 'so potent Art' (1999, V.i.50) of transformation to summon up 'cloud-capp'd towers, the gorgeous palaces, / The solemn temples, the great globe itself' (1999, IV.i.151–2). In the end, that polymath master cook and his abilities are not so far removed from the magician Prospero's.

Works Cited

Ashley, B., J. Hollows, S. Jones, and B. Taylor. 2004. *Food and Cultural Studies*. London. Routledge.

Beaumont, F., and J. Fletcher. 1966–85. *Dramatic Works in the Beaumont & Fletcher Canon*. 6 vols. Ed. F. Bowers. Cambridge. Cambridge University Press.

Brome, R. 1658. *The Lovesick Court*. London. A. Crook.

Chapman, G. 1961. *The Plays of George Chapman*. 2 vols. Ed. T. M. Parrott. New York. Routledge, Kegan & Paul.

Chaucer, Geoffrey. 1962. *The Works of Geoffrey Chaucer*. Ed. W. W. Skeat. Oxford. Oxford University Press.

Cleveland, J. 1910. 'Ode to Ben Jonson upon his ode to Himself'. Ed. F. E. Schelling. London. Dent.

Dalby, A. 1996. *Siren Feasts*. London. Routledge.

Davenant, William. 1968. *The Works of Sir William Davenant*. 2 vols. Facsimile reprint. New York. Blom.

Day, J., W. Rowley, and G. Wilkins. 1995. *Three Renaissance Travel Plays*, inc. *The Travels of the Three English Brothers*. Ed. A. Parr. Manchester. Manchester University Press.

Descartes, René. 1968. *Discourse on Method and other Writings*. Trans. F. E. Sutcliffe. Harmondsworth. Penguin.

Detienne, M., and J. P. Vernant. 1989. *The Cuisine of Sacrifice among the Greeks*. Chicago, IL. University of Chicago Press.

Florio, J. 1598. *A Worlde of Wordes*. London. [A Hatfield] for E. Blount.

Foakes, R. A., and R. T. Rickert, eds. 1961. *Henslowe's Diary*. Cambridge. Cambridge University Press.

Gosson, Stephen. 1579. *The Schoole of Abuse*. London. [T. Dawson] for Thomas Woodcocke.

Greene, R. 1592. *A Groatsworth of Witte*. London. W. Wright.

Hensman, B. 1974. *The Shares of Fletcher, Field & Massinger in Twelve Plays of the Beaumont & Fletcher Canon*. 2 vols. Salzburg. Edwin Mellen Press.

Holinshed, Raphael. 1587. *Chronicles: The First and Second Volumes*. London. Henry Denham.

Jeanneret, Michel. 1991. *A Feast of Words*. Ed. and trans. J. Whiteley and E. Hughes. Chicago, IL. University of Chicago Press.

Jonson, Ben. 1981–82. *The Complete Plays of Ben Jonson*. 4 vols. Ed. G. A. Wilkes. Oxford. Oxford University Press.

Lévi-Strauss, Claude. 1981. *The Raw and the Cooked*. Trans. J. and D. Weightman. London. Jonathan Cape.

Lowe, J. C. B. 1985. 'Cooks in Plautus'. *Classical Antiquity*. 4.1.72–102.

Massinger, Philip. 1964. *A New Way to Pay Old Debts*. Ed. T. W. Craik. London. Ernest Benn.

May, Robert. 1665. *The Accomplisht Cook*. London. [R.Wood] for N. Brooke.

Middleton, Thomas. 1982. *The Old Law*. Ed. C. M. Shaw. London. Garland.

Miles, Rosalind. 1986. *Ben Jonson: His Life and Work*. London. Routledge.

Moryson, Fynes. 1617. *An Itinerary*. London. J. Beale.

Orgel, S. 1981. 'What is a text?' *Research Opportunities in Renaissance Drama*. 24. 3–6.

Ryan, K. 1999. *Shakespeare: The Last Plays*. London. Longman.

Scodel, R. 1993. *Tragic Sacrifice and Menandrian Cooking*. Ann Arbor. University of Michigan Press.

Shakespeare, William. 1999. *The Tempest*. Ed. V. M. and A. T. Vaughan. Walton-on-Thames. Arden/Nelson.

Sidney, Sir Philip. 1989. *Sir Philip Sidney (The Defence of Poesy)*. Ed. K. Duncan-Jones. Oxford. Oxford University Press.

Stallybrass, S., and A. White. 1986. *The Politics and Poetics of Transgression*. London. Methuen.

Strong, Roy. 2002. *Feast: A History of Grand Eating*. London. Jonathan Cape.

Suckling, Sir John. 1971. *The Works of Sir John Suckling*. 2 vols. Ed. T. Clayton and L. Beaurline. Oxford. Clarendon Press.

Vasari, Georgio. 1987. *The Lives of the Artists*. Trans. G. Bull. Harmondsworth. Penguin Books.

Wells, S. 2006. *Shakespeare & Co*. London. Penguin.

Wigg, J. 1991. *The Tudor Kitchens: Hampton Court Palace*. High Wycombe. E. J. Assoc.

Wilkins, J. 2001. *The Boastful Chef*. Oxford. Oxford University Press.

Williamson, J. 1978. *Decoding Advertisements: Ideology and Meaning in Advertising*. London. Boyars.

Wrangham, Richard. 2009. *Catching Fire: How Cooking Made us Human*. New York. Basic Books.

Index